THE
WHOLE
HEALTH
DIET

THE WHOLE HEALTH DIET

A Transformational Approach to Weight Loss

MARK MINCOLLA

JEREMY P. TARCHER / PENGUIN
an imprint of Penguin Random House
New York

JEREMY P. TARCHER/PENGUIN
An imprint of Penguin Random House LLC
375 Hudson Street
New York, New York 10014

Most Tarcher/Penguin books are available at special quantity discounts for bulk purchase for sales promotions, premiums, fund-raising, and educational needs. Special books or book excerpts also can be created to fit specific needs. For details, write: SpecialMarkets@penguinrandomhouse.com.

Library of Congress Cataloging-in-Publication Data

Names: Mincolla, Mark Dana, author.
Title: The whole health diet : a transformational approach to weight loss / Mark Mincolla.
Description: New York: Jeremy P. Tarcher/Penguin, [2015]
Identifiers: LCCN 2015039343 | ISBN 978-0-399-17415-5 (paperback)
Subjects: LCSH: Reducing diets—popular works. | Weight loss—Alternative treatment—Popular works. | Health—Popular works. | Nutrition—Popular works. | Mental healing—Popular works. | Holistic medicine. | BISAC: BODY, MIND & SPIRIT/Healing/Energy (Chi Kung, Reiki, Polarity). | HEALTH & FITNESS/Diets. | HEALTH & FITNESS/Alternative Therapies.
Classification: LCC RM222.2 .M527 2015 | DDC 613.2/5—dc23
LC record available at http://lccn.loc.gov/2015039343

Printed in the United States of America
1   3   5   7   9   10   8   6   4   2

BOOK DESIGN BY TANYA MAIBORODA

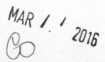

MAR 1 1 2016

This book is dedicated to Albert Einstein,
for awakening the world from its Newtonian slumber.

CONTENTS

INTRODUCTION

I often describe myself as a holistic problem solver. I've performed tens of thousands of nutritional therapy consultations—in both the private and corporate sectors—over the past three decades and have managed to successfully solve a majority of the health care problems I've been confronted with. Unfortunately, many of the patients that I've counseled arrive at my doorstep only after the medical orthodoxy has given up on them. Sadly, my office is all too often "the last stop."

They've come to me seeking nutritional assistance for heart disease, type 2 diabetes, Parkinson's disease, irritable bowel syndrome, attention deficit/hyperactivity disorder—the list goes on. Not so surprisingly, many of them are overweight when I first see them. Rarely, if ever, have I put any of them on formal weight loss diets, yet, oddly enough, a vast majority of them lose the weight they need to, and manage to keep it off.

My commitment has always been to help patients attain and maintain vitality by teaching them to cultivate some modicum of holistic integrity, and to save a life whenever possible. I've always operated under the assumption that if I can help people to achieve balance in body, mind, and spirit, I will have put them in the best position to heal what ails them. As far as dealing with patients who suffer from being overweight and from obesity, my philosophy and approach have always been exactly the same. To my way of thinking, these problems are the natural result of a lifestyle that's devoid of holism. The only real antidote for these afflictions is a commitment to conscious living and a dedication to cultivating balance in body, mind, and spirit. It will never be about calorie-counting diet fads. Truth be told, it's about holistic transformation—optimal nutrition, emotional freedom, and spiritual sentience.

Meanwhile, as America gourmandizes on empty calories, amasses incalculable pounds, and sabotages its collective body, mind, and spirit, it becomes increasingly desperate for effectual solutions. And as it continues its desperate search for answers, it exposes its aggregate predilection for false promise and specious, push-button solutions that don't work. Moreover, there is some question as to which worriment is worse—its addiction to food or its obsession with spurious solutions. There seems to be no end to America's "purple pill" mentality. We appear insistent on clinging to the notion that the next quick fix is "the one." Meanwhile, the knaves are lined up at our door and, as always, they're all too willing to take advantage of our desperation and gullibility. We continue to exhibit a high tolerance for their spin, in spite of the fact that their sham solutions remain infinitely ineffectual.

The cold, hard truth is if we're ever to resolve this dreadful dilemma, we must first be willing to dig down deeper. The diet du jour cannot solve this problem. We're not gaining weight simply because we're eating too much. We're eating too much because we're broken. We've become so averse to feeling the pain at the root of our "dis-ease" that we're now driven to distraction with food. Weight loss dieting alone cannot get to the bottom of this problem. If our failed history of dieting tells us anything about solving this problem, it's that it is time for us to stop "mowing the weeds."

Our current pandemic weight problem is representative of a disease that's causally rooted in dis-ease. Anything short of a wholehearted commitment to heal ourselves in body, mind, and spirit will merely result in more failure, and the only thing that we'll lose is more money.

The Whole Health Diet is the antidieting diet plan. It's very much about state-of-the-art, optimal nutrition, but it's also about arriving at your ideal weight as the natural result of attaining and maintaining your holistic balance. The WHD escorts the reader through a profound shift in consciousness. By adroitly making the connection between weight and metabolism, emotion, nutrition, physiology, brain (mind) neurology, and spirituality, the WHD provides the reader with the details of "how to" attain true holistic balance and wellness. I believe that by doing so, it's providing the only real solution to the problem of overweight/obesity.

The WHD addresses the unpopular truth about weight gain and obesity. Based on the belief that we are living in a time of great transformation, this means people are at last ready to hear the truth about this problem. The WHD starts with the idea that this problem is representative of a disease that is causally rooted in the dis-ease of the human heart.

Dis-ease is to disease what a droplet is to a flood. Every disturbing emotion that trickles to the heart flows until it overflows. So it is with this distressing problem. Obesity and being overweight are the clear results of overeating, but the real hunger problem is in the heart.

It's not hard to understand why so many Americans are currently overweight and obese from food addiction. In today's world, hearts are broken early and often. Our personal and cultural pains run deep. We're living our lives at such a breakneck pace that we no longer have any time for our deeper emotional needs to matter. For many, the more ceaseless the stress, the more that love and peace become a distant memory.

As we awaken each day to reports of a slumping global economy, human rights violations, and the growing threat of terrorism, we're constantly reminded that we're living in a world of great uncertainty. Stress, depression, anxiety, confusion, pain, and suffering have all become part of our de-evolutionary norm.

The greater our pain and suffering, the stronger is our drive to seek pleasure. The more we hurt, the more we eat. The more we eat, the greater our likelihood of gaining weight. The false promise of fad weight loss dieting only serves to further the confusion, pain, and suffering. Most of these bogus weight loss programs are nothing more than serpentine revenue machines, designed to feed off of the desperate. As far as the few legitimate programs that do exist, most are simply not equipped to support their respective dieters in the attainment and maintenance of their holistic balance, and far fewer of them still are capable of providing the proper guidance and inspiration necessary to help them rise above their dysfunctional relationship with food.

This conflicting cycle of feeling out of control, overeating, gaining weight, never really understanding why, and then rushing into the next new fad diet program is positively ruinous. If we are ever to experience the true lasting results we so deserve, we'll need to start looking much deeper. In order for our solutions to be more effective, they will have to take us much deeper.

The Whole Health Diet plan represents a radical departure from the flawed mind-set of fad dieting. My previous book *Whole Health* boldly and clearly spells out a plan to empower readers to attain true wellness and balance—asserting that in so doing they will, in time, naturally gravitate to their ideal weight. In short, the present book asserts that it's only by maintaining a holistically balanced lifestyle, with the assistance of quantum energy healing practices, that this problem can be permanently solved. If we are to turn the key that opens the door beyond the threshold to a place of new possibilities, we'll have to put aside our natural resistance to change.

We're living in a time of great change. Everything is reformatting; everything including us. Who we are—how we live, love, and heal—is currently in a state of great flux. We are in the midst of an identity crisis of unparalleled proportions. This season of change is a time of deepening for us all. Many of our mechanistic systems and theories are now becoming obsolete. They are anachronistic solutions equipped to deal with problems from a different time. From the material perspective everything appears to be the same, but based on what we've learned from the 2011 Nobel Prize–winning research of Saul Perlmutter, Adam G. Riess, and Brian P. Schmidt, the universe is expanding at an accelerated rate. Thus, our energy and the energy of everything around us is now vibrating at a significantly higher frequency than ever before. Never before have our minds been so filled with thought, our hearts so swollen with emotion, and our spirits so effulgent with quantum possibility. Our perceptions of reality and baselines for possibility are being superconsciously reformatted. The fading illusion of a structurally supportive, three-dimensional reality and five-sensory absoluteness is literally dematerializing. The classical is giving way to the quantum. As we awaken to this energy-based reality, we're beginning to discover that we're far more than mere material beings, bound by corporeal limitation. Rather, we are multidimensional energy beings with an infinite capacity for extrasensory possibility.

Our once-predictable material world—and all that it programmed us to accept as possible—is suddenly undergoing sweeping changes. Once governed by the material parameters of classical mechanics, our understanding of science, health care, nutrition, and life in general has been forever altered as we've been invited to take a quantum leap into the void.

The energetic frequencies that emanate from within our expeditiously evolving minds and hearts are now vibrating at an extraordinary pace. The rapid expansion of each human microcosm is part of an infinite cause-and-effect loop. We are both the receivers and the transmitters of radical change. The cosmos is changing, and we are the cosmos. Never before have we thought so much, dreamed so much, felt so much, and done so much. And as much as we're doing today, we'll do even more tomorrow. With all the repercussive demands and growing pains associated with this expansion, our list of needs also grows ever longer. We'll need more love, care, healing, and understanding. We'll also need more energy to emanate from our love, care, healing, and understanding—because as our light expands, tension from any darkness will be released. As our personal growing pains intensify, our healing systems are forced to keep pace.

Now any medicine that comes solely in the form of the blade or the pill is no longer sufficient. At last the doctor's touch is as important (if not *more* important) than either. Moreover, any physicians who fail to understand that both they and their patients are not merely anatomical beings, but multidimensional beings with vital energy needs, will simply be outmoded. Furthermore, any patients who fail to engage in holistic, bioenergetic disease prevention will remain bound and trussed to a life of chronic disease and pharmaceutical dependency.

Our future is arriving at last, and as the revised picture of health care gradually unfolds before us, it will continue to reveal a very different sort of image from what any of us might have ever imagined. We'll find that it's not about neoteric machinery, space-age technology, or state-of-the-art chemistry. In fact, it will no longer be based on mechanistic principles. More and more, we'll see that the new burgeoning age of health care will be about the exploration of the *vital life force* and the extrasensory potential of human energy. You and I are about to become our own physicians, and we'll soon see that we've always possessed the miracle medicine that we've long been waiting for, within our own energy field. And we'll also soon discover that once whole, we will no longer have to lose weight over and over again. For, after having attained the lasting fulfillment of holistic balance, we'll no longer feel driven to fill ourselves full.

CHAPTER 1

OVERWEIGHT, OBESE, AND DYING TO BE TRANSFORMED

The Scope of the Problem

According to the World Health Organization, 3.4 million people globally are dying each year from being overweight or obese.[1] Studies show that being chronically overweight and/or obese significantly increases the risk of type 2 diabetes, cancer, lung disease, kidney disease, sleep apnea, osteoarthritis, fatty liver disease, and depression. Moreover, some research even reveals significant health risks associated with being moderately or slightly overweight.

For example, in 2004 Frank Hu of the Harvard School of Public Health authored a study in which 115,000 women ages thirty to fifty-five were followed for nearly a decade, and those who were as little as 5 percent overweight were 30 percent more likely to develop heart disease.[2] Those women who were only mildly to moderately overweight incurred a risk of heart disease 80 percent higher than that of their counterparts. Those women who were 30 percent or more overweight were 300 percent more likely to develop heart disease.

One in three adults worldwide are currently overweight or obese. One widely accepted medical definition of obesity is a five foot, nine inch adult who weighs over 202 pounds. According to the Centers for Disease Control and Prevention, 69 percent of Americans are overweight and 35 percent are obese, burdening the nation with an annual health care cost of $150 billion.[3] Moreover, experts say that a majority of U.S. residents will be obese by the end of the next two decades, with obesity rates as high as 60 percent in as many as thirteen states by the year 2030. To date there are no effective, long-term solutions. Hundreds of millions of Americans diet continuously, spending tens of billions of dollars on weight loss each year, yet according to most studies conducted over the past fifty years, approximately 95 percent of all diets fail within the first year and less than 3 percent of people who take weight off keep it off for at least five years.

The CDC employs body mass index (BMI) as the standard for determining degrees of overweight and obesity. BMI is the measurement of body fat based on height and weight. It is calculated by dividing weight in pounds by height in inches squared times a factor of 703.

There are a number of reliable Internet sites that can help with BMI computation. A BMI of 18.5 or lower is considered underweight. A BMI of 18.6 to 24.9 represents the norm. A BMI of 25 to 29.9 is overweight, and a BMI of 30 or higher is considered obese. According to a recent study performed by the London School of Hygiene and Tropical Medicine, which calculated the average

BMIs of 177 countries, the United States has the fifth highest BMI in the world. Here's a sampling of some national BMI averages for comparison:[4]

Japan 21.93
China 22.86
Italy 23.49
France 23.56
Spain 24.52
Germany 25.32
United Kingdom 26.19
United States 27.82

In spite of the recent deluge of diet theories and fad weight loss programs, our national BMI average continues to rise.

The average American now weighs twenty-three pounds more than his or her ideal body weight. With two-thirds of America now overweight or obese, the perception regarding the average body type is shifting as well. Studies that have looked at our changing attitudes about being overweight are beginning to show that younger generations of overweight Americans are now starting to perceive themselves as part of a healthy norm. "It's quite clear that people are changing their idea of what an acceptable body size is," says Nicholas Christakis of Harvard Medical School. "As the average body weight goes up, there's more acceptance of heavier body types. This, in turn, clears the path for even more people to put on weight."[5]

Our culture now perceives being overweight as being part of the norm.

Over the past fifty years ours has become a "supersized" and "special-sized" culture, custom designed to facilitate the emerging "bigger body" trend. We've been steadily increasing the portion sizes of the fast foods and sugary beverages sold in restaurants, movie theaters, sports arenas, malls, food carts, and delis over the past two generations. Prior to the late 1960s, the largest soda sold at any fast food counter was only seven ounces, which pales in comparison to today's sixty-four-ounce "Double Gulp."

We've created more spacious seating options for virtually all of our public transportation systems, theaters, theme park rides, and stadiums. Our gurneys, operating tables, ambulances, and coffin sizes have all become much wider and longer as well. Over the past fifty years America has gradually adapted itself to being larger. Worse, being overweight has become such a cultural norm, the mind-set is now embedded in our younger generation.

The population of overweight children in the United States is growing at a disturbingly accelerated rate, as one-third of our children are now considered overweight or obese. This represents a statistical tripling over the past forty years. Obesity has moved ahead of drug abuse and tobacco as the current number-one health concern among parents in the United States.

Childhood obesity is responsible for a wide range of serious health problems once common only in adults, such as elevated cholesterol and high blood pressure. Kids' health problems caused by being overweight or obese are likely to be lifelong and, in some cases, life threatening. Perhaps the dire nature of this tragedy was best summarized by former surgeon general Richard Carmona when he said, "Because of the increasing rates of obesity, unhealthy eating habits, and physical inactivity, you may see the first generation that will be less healthy and have a shorter life expectancy than their parents."[6]

Kids have become considerably more sedentary, now spending 90 percent of their free time in front of a computer screen, playing video games, or watching television. Today's busy family has considerably less time to shop for and prepare healthy, home-cooked meals. Time constraints, virtual lifestyle, and palate programming are among the many influences that are seeding the next generation of overweight, obese, and unhealthy Americans. It's clear that we're speeding headlong into a disaster, with no rescue plan.

Currently, there are more than a hundred popular dietary theories, most of which contradict each other—and none of which have proven particularly effective. Proponents of each insist that successful weight loss can be negotiated by simply following a diet program aligned with its code. For instance, one theory promotes following the fifteen-thousand-year-old diet of your Paleolithic ancestors, claiming that it's naturally synchronized with your gene map. Another theory subscribes to the premise that you can best maximize your nutritional efficiency by consuming those foods that are aligned with your blood type. There are many similar such theories that are based on the diets of Okinawans, French women, Hindus, and Buddhists.

According to the Food Addiction Institute, most diets have a success rate of between 10 and 30 percent.[7]

Weight Watchers is widely believed to be the most successful diet program in the world today. Expert estimations of their success rate are between 5 and 10 percent. Despite such failure rates, diet programs continue to attract droves of new and repeat dieters.

Nearly one-third of our entire nation takes up dieting every year. According to ongoing research, fad dieting simply doesn't work. Moreover, studies show that a majority of dieters who buy into the latest fad diets each year are increasingly likely to be among the "serial dieter" population. Considering these disheartening facts, one can only arrive at the conclusion that fad diets are not designed for the benefit of the dieter. Fad diets are designed for the benefit of their designers. There's no doubt that we have a very serious and costly problem on our hands, for which there is presently no viable solution.

Among the many reasons why diets don't work is that they're based on an overly simplistic, one-size-fits-all theory and they fail to address the deeper emotional roots of overeating behaviors. In order to have any real hope of solving this grave problem, we'll need to start thinking out of the box—thinking more broadly and much deeper about our broken selves, and our attraction to being fixed by food.

Most of our current metabolic problem-solving models are based on physical, calorie-counting strategies. They clearly don't work. They fail to take into account the fact that besides being material, physical beings, humans are also composed of subtle mental, emotional, and spiritual energies. Truth be told, our minds, emotions, and spirits all play a significant role in shaping the human behaviors that profoundly influence our relationship with food.

The calorie-counting approach to fixing this problem is merely a reflection of a fading, decades-old way of thinking. We've been programmed by our mechanistic, cultural downloading to think and problem-solve in overly simplistic material terms. When it comes to tackling the problem of an increasing overweight and obese population, so much mental, emotional, and spiritual energy lies at the core that there can be no lasting relief provided by mere calorie counting.

Today, we lead exceedingly stressful existences. Our day-to-day anxieties have never been so paralyzing. The greater the pressure, the more mentally, emotionally, and spiritually reactive we become. The more reactive we become, the more susceptible we are to the quick fix—and a good food fix is never far away.

More than ever before, we're in need of more "whole solutions"—solutions that address the mind, emotion, and spirit, not just the body. The present solutions are doing us absolutely no earthly good. In fact, they're fast becoming part of the problem. It's time we stopped changing our diets and started transforming our consciousness.

University of Missouri researchers recently discovered that a non-diet, "Eat for Life" approach, one that focuses on a conscious, intuitive lifestyle and eating habits, is far more effective than traditional weight loss programs at improving body image and decreasing eating disorders. The focus of this study was to get subjects more tuned in to their own bodies and minds—to get them to become more familiar with their own internal physical, emotional, and mental cues for hunger and fullness rather than calorie counting and weighing on scales.

An Obsolete Problem-Solving Mentality

Fad dieting hasn't yet, nor will it ever, solve the problem of a chronic overweight and obese America. It reflects decades of erroneous thinking and corrupt intentions. Moreover, it reveals an antiquated, matter-based mentality that can't really solve *any* problems very well, because matter doesn't even exist.

As author Daniel Quinn explains in *Ishmael*, we are all captives of "a story Mother Culture is telling us." Our culture has been stuck in a time warp for nearly a century now. We can't seem to escape the ancient Aristotelian world of solid forms. Everything we believe we can and can't do—the scope of all our problems and our problem-solving potential—is based on an obsolete perception of reality. And so, based on this flawed, matter-based thinking, millions of people around the world will once again count their caloric intake today, take a brisk walk around the block, and jump on the scale in hopes of losing weight. Ours remains a world of solid forms insistent on hanging on for dear life to the dictates of a bygone Newtonian era.

Sir Isaac Newton first published his *Philosophiae Naturalis Principia Mathematica* on July 5, 1687. In this work Newton formulated the laws of motion, gravity, and classical mechanics that would shape our view of the physical universe for more than three hundred years. By expounding on the interrelationship between the physical concepts of force, mass, and acceleration, Newtonian mechanics laid the foundations for matter-centric thinking. Matter then was believed to be the binding substance that held the universe together. For the better part of three centuries, and still even today, matter-based reality continues to remain the standard by which we live, love, learn, and problem-solve. During the first part of the twentieth century a new and very different story of reality would start to emerge thanks in part to the likes of Max Planck, Albert Einstein, and Werner Heisenberg.

Max Planck, a Nobel Prize–winning physicist and the founder of quantum theory, was among the first paradigm-shifting scientists to awaken the world to the reality that matter doesn't exist. Planck said, "There is no matter as such. All matter originates and exists only by virtue of a force which brings the particles of an atom to vibration and holds this most minute solar system of the atom together. We must assume behind this force the existence of a conscious and intelligent mind. This mind is the matrix of all matter."[8] He emphasized that matter is but a mirage, and that the energy of consciousness is, in fact, the true binding substance of the universe. Planck remains a central figure in the consciousness shift to a more energy-centric reality. His work profoundly inspired and ultimately influenced the work of Albert Einstein.

In his groundbreaking theory of relativity, Einstein reinforced an emerging reality that was based on energy rather than matter—a reality in which the perceptible is continually created by the imperceptible. When he was awarded the Nobel Prize in 1921, the world was suddenly forced to acknowledge that the universe was composed of 99.999 percent energy.

In 1932, Werner Heisenberg was awarded his Nobel Prize in Physics for discovering a way to formulate quantum mechanics in understandable matrices.

In the span of one generation, reality as we'd known it had been turned upside down. Après Planck, Einstein, and Heisenberg, reality would never be the same. Tables, chairs, and people like you and me—once thought of as solid material objects—were now understood as masses of imperceptible energy governed by very different laws. A world and universe once seen as solid ice cubes was now more like flowing water. The centuries-old classical mechanics of Aristotle and Sir Isaac Newton were at once supplanted by a quantum view. Reality would never be the same, but it would take quite a while for our minds to grasp the fact.

Astonishingly enough, nearly a century after Einstein's theory of relativity, the prevailing perception of reality in our world continues to center on the laws of Newton's classical mechanics, material biology, and five-sensory perception. In fact, all the hierarchies that currently govern our way of life are still materially based. For example, the material hierarchy that presently sets the standard for our practice of medicine, nutrition, and weight loss progresses from cell, to tissue, to organ, and finally to organism. It somehow manages to ignore all the hierarchical elements that precede the cell, namely molecules, atoms, and particles. All but disregarding the Nobel-winning work of Planck, Einstein, and Heisenberg, our world remains insistent on reducing an energy-based cosmos down to its five-sensory level of understanding. We continue to cling to the belief that life begins at the cellular level. We're material beings, our food is composed of material properties, and the only way we can effectively lose weight is by reducing material calories. We've got to get over our Newtonian hangover!

Matter doesn't exist. Everything is energy, including you, me, and the foods we eat. But we don't have to take a quantum leap to wrap our heads around this stuff. There are much simpler ways of looking at it. For example, we're abundantly aware of the potential health effects of negative thoughts and emotions. Our thoughts and emotions are imperceptible energies that elude our five senses, yet they're more than capable of imposing dramatic effects on our material cells. Some recent studies have shown that a great deal of our chronic overweight and obesity problem is directly related to negative thoughts and feelings. We must remember that everything is energy. Thoughts and feelings are energies, as are the foods we eat. Our practice of medicine, nutrition, and weight loss can be energetically adapted to meet our present weight loss needs with far greater efficiency.

I've worked with thousands of patients over the past three decades, and together we've repeatedly demonstrated the remarkable healing and weight loss potential of energy. Drawing from quantum theory, the Whole Health Diet presents effective energy-healing applications that exceed the limitations of the present matter-based problem-solving approaches to health care and weight loss. Before learning about these remarkable energy-healing applications, we'll have to first change our thinking and expand our awareness.

A Shift in Awareness

Classical, matter-based thinking would have us believe that the only way to lose weight is through diet and exercise. While there's little question as to whether or not this is true, the data tell us that it's likely to be true for only a short while. Based on my years of experience, one reason why most diets fail within the first year is because energy, typically in the form of human emotion, ultimately gets in the way. Our conscious mind represents the logical thinking center within us that makes the New Year's resolution to lose weight and join a health club, but this part of our mind has only enough muscle to process two thousand bits of information per second. Neuroplasticity research (Dr. Richard Davidson) has established this as the rate at which the conscious mind processes information. A bit represents a mathematical parameter affecting the mind's processing of information. Our unconscious mind, representing our storehouse of emotional memories, mostly negative, can process up to four hundred billion bits of information per second. Quantum, energy-based thinking tells us that if we really marshaled the powerful energy of our mental intention we could lose weight by simply manifesting the pounds off.

There: I give you a moment to pick up your book, which I'm quite certain just fell to the floor.

According to the laws of quantum mechanics, consciously directed intent is capable of altering the behavior of the fundamental concepts that appear to us as matter. But this isn't any "ready-access, push-button" stuff here. This requires a significant change of mind.

Quantum, energy-based thinking may be directed only from our superconscious mind. Only superconsciousness has access to the quantum energy matrix—a thought domain of unlimited manifest power. Now the time has come for us to open the door to this mind state of infinite possibility. But before we do, we first need to understand a bit more about the transformational shift that's leading us there. Many aren't aware of it, but we are currently undergoing a collective shift in consciousness. This shift is nature's way of expanding awareness as part of a greater cosmic evolutionary growth.

In the world of energy, change is natural. As Einstein would remind us, energy is always in a state of flux. Energy could be defined as power in motion—motion generated by vibrating particles that produce wave frequency. Waves rise as the result of amassing energy, ultimately reaching a crescendo. Once the wave hits its peak it begins to release energy as it decays, ultimately giving way to a new cycle. All the energy in the universe progresses through this cycle of beginning, middle, end, and new beginning. The wave is therefore a perfect metaphor for understanding the present cosmic shift. Everything, including us, is in a constant state of change, and our present changes are swift and dramatic. Every facet of our existence has been in an ascending wave cycle and is now fast approaching a tipping point. It's as if everything in our lives has been sped up and intensified—everything including (and especially) our problems. While the world news headlines have never been particularly good, they have never been quite so bad.

At the time I was writing this book, Israelis and Palestinians were at war in the Gaza Strip, Pro-Russian rebels had shot down a commercial airliner over the Ukraine, Syrian troops had advanced on rebels in a contested Damascus suburb, a powerful earthquake had killed hundreds in southern China, Islamic terrorists in Iraq had killed Christian children and buried Christian refugees alive, and there was rioting in the streets in Ferguson, Missouri. The world has always been in turmoil, but nothing quite like this. Problems that have always been bad appear to be worsening.

One of the many ways in which our problems as a species manifest themselves is in our worsening national obesity dilemma. In 1985, America had an adult obesity rate of 15 percent. Today the rate has risen to nearly 30 percent, almost doubling over the past thirty years. As is true with every aspect of nature, the cosmos will ultimately cleanse itself from the rising tensions of negative energies. As when low pressure and pollution build up in the atmosphere, nature's response is a good hard cleansing rain. If ever there was a need for a transformational cleansing of human consciousness, it would be right now. More than ever we need to hit the reset button in our minds in order to transcend our present transgressions.

For many of us, any change is disorienting. This prospect of radical change will probably seem overwhelming to some. Though we're not likely aware of it, the gradual changes that are a part of a greater transformation are taking place in our lives even as I write this—it's just difficult to notice because it's all unfolding incrementally and unsuspectingly.

Every day for what may seem like an eternity, we wake up at the same time, drink the same coffee, eat the same breakfast, kiss the same lover on the same lips, pull the same car out of the same garage, and drive the same route to the same workplace. Then one day out of the blue, we have a stunning revelation that the relationship or job we've had for years is simply no longer aligned with our changing needs. Suddenly our reality is transformed, and our whole world is turned upside down. Although it may be difficult for us to pinpoint, our radical life shift is likely prompted by a series of subtle shifts in our thinking that have taken place gradually over the course of time. This long-term, incremental cause-and-effect process represents how transformation manifests from an energy perspective. In the world of energy, change may be best described as an infinite cycling of causes and effects, ultimately amassing to transformational tipping points and resulting in a higher level of action.

Change is constantly happening around us, within us, and through us. It's a symbiotic process. All forces great and small are forever influencing and being influenced by each other's changes, as together they drive each other closer to transformation and a more evolved action. It's transformational thinking that opens the door to the quantum matrix of infinite possibilities. By thinking bigger thoughts, we cultivate the kind of mind-set that allows us to rise above our ever-evolving problems. But we have to be willing to stretch our minds.

We've been weaned on finite material—thoughts about things like coffee cups, breakfasts, good-bye kisses, and getting to work on time. But when it comes to the quantum transformation of our mind, everything—especially the prospect of possibilities—becomes infinitely expansive. Remember, in the world of energy, there is constant change perpetuated by symbiotic cause and effect. We are all presently shifting into quantum consciousness, in part because of influences from surrounding energies. The higher the energy frequencies that we're linked to, the more expansive will be our changes, and the more expansive our changes, the more powerful our transformational shifting. It's like a game of quantum cause-and-effect Ping-Pong—and it's presently playing out with great speed and intensity. Yesterday's "future shock," in which too much change happened in too short a period of time, has simply become today's "transformational shift." Our thinking has been sped up and intensified by all the events surrounding us.

I was utterly astounded to hear that scientists from NASA reported that there are approximately 150 million Earth-like planets, likely capable of facilitating life, within our own galaxy alone. I couldn't help but think about all the truly astonishing changes that now take place during the course of a single lifetime. I also thought about how mightily they've contributed both figuratively and literally to the reshaping of our expanding minds.

We are all part of an interconnected circle of life that manifests cycles of perpetual movement and changes. This ever-evolving energy loop extends from self to family, neighborhood, community, city, state, nation, continent, planet, solar system, galaxy, universe, multiverse, cosmos, and back to self. And though it may be our inclination to think locally, all our changes and transformations are directly tied to a constant flow of ever-changing events that extend from far beyond the orbit of our mundane, terrestrial existence. The cosmos to which we are inextricably bound is forever changing its form. With each of our thoughts and actions we influence everything that happens in the infinite distances beyond, just as their energies return to influence our evolving changes. If energy drives change, symbiosis shapes it. This "bigger picture" perspective is in evidence everywhere in nature. You don't have to look very far to see the energy-based power of cosmic interconnectedness.

Imagine, if you will, a large hurricane system extending over a two-thousand-mile area. Such a system would surely impose life-changing and life-threatening effects on many thousands of people, places, and things in a number of global regions for a great many days. Also, imagine the far-reaching cataclysmic potential of a solar flare. Solar flares, or magnetic storms, occur when extremely high concentrations of energy that have built up in the solar atmosphere are suddenly released. Solar flare radiation is emitted across the entire electromagnetic spectrum, capable of sending shockwaves through the core of the Earth, causing extensive blackouts and dramatically altering communications networks. And since humans are electromagnetic beings, solar flares have even been shown to affect our thoughts, emotions, behaviors, and our physical health.

Every form of energy in the cosmos is engaged in an endless dance of cause and effect—the music has never been so loud and our dance steps have never been so frenzied. This present cosmic season of change is one of great turbulence. You can't help but feel that something very different is in the air, as the magnitude and scope of our problems are far greater than ever before. Take a good look deep within and all around you. Look at yourself, your family, friends, neighborhood, community, nation, and world. Everywhere you look, there are serious problems. Problems like never before. Most of what were once our most effective problem-solving strategies have at once been rendered powerless.

The magnitude of our current obesity problem has at last become so panoptic that instead of turning to yet another dietary solution, we now need to start looking at the fundamental flaw in ourselves—our thinking and our consciousness. As our problems continue to amass energy, it's time for us to match their destructive force with a more highly evolved problem-solving power. At the risk of overstating the obvious, we can't hope to solve space shuttle problems with a horse-and-buggy mentality. As long as we insist on employing the same inefficacious, timeworn solutions, this dilemma will only continue to worsen.

The real solution to this problem begins with the transformation of our thinking. The present solutions are both ineffectual and corrupt, as they fail to equip, empower, and inspire the dieter for any lasting success, choosing instead to capitalize on their desperation and vulnerability.

Calorie-counting fad diets come and go, continuing to find new ways to feed us the same old "leftovers" with a new spin. And while the angles of their spin may appeal to our curiosity, they're simply putting a different color lipstick on the same old pig. Regardless of whether they're evoking the Bible, South Beach, or Hollywood, they're just leading us down the same old tired, worn path to nowhere.

Imagine

The WHD challenges us to transform our anachronistic, matter-based consciousness—to eradicate our self-limited thinking and to envision ourselves as problem solvers with total access to a matrix of infinite possibility.

Imagine awakening to the newly discovered awareness that half your life story is unrealized. Imagine making the stunning discovery that there's a quantum, extrasensory reality that stretches far beyond the five-sensory biological programming that's been obstructing your panorama. Imagine exercising your extrasensory power for the first time and finding out that your power is capable of transforming your life, your health, your metabolism, and your weight loss potential. Imagine discovering that you can regulate the emotion, mood, and thought energies that affect your eating behavior and your calorie-burning potential. Imagine learning that you and every one of the seven billion people you share the planet with have a unique energy signature, similar to DNA. Imagine that each and every form of food on the planet also has its own unique energy signature. Your energy DNA is different from your neighbor's, and blueberries have an energy DNA that's different from strawberries'. Imagine that there is an easy-to-learn system that can effectively help you determine how to balance your energy DNA with the energies of all the foods you eat so as to help you burn calories with maximum efficiency. Finally, imagine that there is a personalized diet system for you and you alone that enables you to optimize your health and maximize your weight loss potential by holistically balancing all your life force energy.

As you are about to discover, the Whole Health Diet is just such a system.

Transformational Solutions for
Weight Gain and Obesity

The WHD presents you with a holistic, bioenergetic approach to metabolic weight loss management. This book goes on to tackle the problems of weight gain associated with emotional eating (i.e., addiction), but the thing that separates the WHD from all other diet plans is its time-tested, energy-based nutritional and metabolic healing protocols. It teaches you how to develop and maintain your own personalized, energy-calibrated nutrition plan. The WHD guides you through a series of lesson plans teaching you how to energetically self-diagnose your glandular calorie-burning potential. This book also shares a number of therapeutic energy exercises that allow you to rebalance your metabolic deficiencies. In addition, you are taught how to electromagnetically test yourself for metabolic food intolerances. By identifying the foods that support and the foods that sabotage your body's calorie-burning potential, you're able to customize a dietary map to follow for greater weight loss efficiency.

Dietary weight loss programs are based solely on cellular matter (cells and calories). Fad diet designers continue to focus their pitches purely on the science of weight loss, failing to take into consideration the importance of life-changing energies. Millions of serial dieters fail to keep weight off not because of calorie reduction failure, but rather because of recurrent, deep-seated, negative emotional and mental thought patterns. The energies generated by these chronic, agonizing patterns assert a physiological influence that can have a profound effect on vital glands and organs, ultimately impairing the potential for optimal weight loss. Subtle energies such as these govern every aspect of our lives, yet because they elude our five senses we've struggled to fully understand them.

Our world is just now beginning to embrace healing energy applications once common only to Eastern culture. Growing numbers of us are turning to acupuncture, acupressure, Reiki, and qigong for healing and weight loss. The centuries-old effectiveness of healing arts such as these validates the presence and emphasizes the vital importance of unseen life force energy.

"Life force energy" is a term representing a concept that has been understood for millennia. It refers to the imperceptible vital essence that embodies all living things, the current of life, and the essence of vitality within all cells, tissues, organs, and organisms. As in my earlier book *Whole Health*, in this book I have devised a series of therapeutic energy protocols intended to assist readers who are striving for greater holistic health. Holistic health equals balanced metabolism, which results in ideal weight.

There are three major components of the WHD's therapeutic energy protocols:

1. SUPERCONSCIOUS ENERGY. Most of our lifetime is spent in conscious and unconscious mental states that reflect our wishing, striving, attaining, and surrendering. That is to say, our mind wishes for certain results that we can then strive for until either we attain them or we decide to surrender. Our conscious mind represents limited attainment power that's generally of a pretty positive nature. Our unconscious mind, on the other hand, represents a far greater force—but of a more defensive, if not subversive, nature.

Everything is energy, even consciousness. The word "energy" implies flux and variability, and so it is with human consciousness—which can be as low as the ocean floor or as elevated as the uppermost regions of the stratosphere. Most of us typically vacillate between an elevated conscious intention, such as a resolution to lose weight, and an unconscious impulse to sabotage such a plan. On any given day, we're likely to come up with 1,000 good intentions and 1,001 reasons not to follow through with them. This is business as usual, with the never-ending battle between our conscious and unconscious mind. Few of us are even aware of this frustrating process, and fewer of us still are aware of the fact that we have the power to actually do something about it. Instead of being randomly dictated to by the vicissitudes of our ever-changing mind, we can choose to lock into a higher thought frequency. It's all about being conscious of our consciousness. This can take us beyond our limited consciousness—the unconscious game of Ping-Pong— to a state of superconscious mind.

Nowadays, superconscious mind is often associated with exceptional human function (EHF). Extraordinary human potentials that defy the known laws of physics are currently being researched by the governments of Russia, China, and the United States. EHF research has scientifically affirmed the infinite latitude of the human mind. Conscious mind is limited. Unconscious mind is defensive. Superconscious mind knows no limitation. This is why the WHD seeks to help you access your superconscious mind. No more yo-yo dieting. No more Ping-Pong mentality. Quantum mechanics has proven that with properly focused intent, you have the superconscious potential to think your weight off. You will discover exactly how to engage the powers of your superconscious mind for the purposes of enhancing your weight loss potential in later chapters.

2. ELECTROMAGNETIC ENERGY. Mother Nature provided us with an extremely efficient and reliable defense system, since one of her top priorities is the survival of our species. Our defense system is principally made up of our intrinsic cardiac ganglia, brain, and nervous system. The intrinsic cardiac ganglia comprise bundles of afferent nerves that, among other things, provide us with extrasensory awareness—awareness that is transmitted bodily by neural electricity. The human body produces about .025 volts of ambient electricity at ten cycles per second. The science of medicine frequently implements scanning methods such as EEGs, EKGs, and MRIs to observe the body's electrical properties for diagnostic purposes. The charge produced by the higher cognition from our intrinsic cardiac ganglia generates a biofeedback response that relays its perceptions via our nervous system and on to our body's global electromagnetic pathways. This electromagnetic response can be implemented for energy-based self-diagnosis, therapeutic balancing, and food intolerance testing.

Over the past three decades I've developed the Whole Health healing and diet plans and perfected their trademark Electromagnetic Muscle Testing system for the express purposes of providing readers with tools to assess organ strengths and weaknesses, identify food intolerances, and engage therapeutic balancing techniques. These electromagnetic energy-based protocols are what separate the WHD from all other diet plans. The EMT techniques elevate the dieting experience far beyond a generalized one-size-fits-all approach. They provide you with the wherewithal to design your own personalized plan and assist you in keeping up with the fluidity of your ever-changing metabolic and nutritional needs. As you will clearly see in the chapters that lie ahead, your electromagnetic energy field is a precious wellspring of accessible information that will help you transform your dieting experience.

3. LIFE FORCE ENERGY (QIGONG AND ENERGY MEDICINE). The energy that animates life and binds the cosmos may elude the five human senses, but its power remains ever available to anyone with enough extrasensory perception, conscious intent, and discipline to master the art of directing it. The Chinese have developed many detailed practices that have enabled them to master the art of directing life force energy for generations.

In Chinese the word *qi* (pronounced "chee"; also spelled *ch'i*) means "energy" and the word *gong* means "mastery." Qigong is an ancient healing art form whose origins are said to go back some three thousand years. The ancient Chinese had an innate understanding of the ways of qi. They instinctually knew that, though imperceptible, qi represented the greatest power in the cosmos. Thus, they developed eight systems of martial arts and healing arts to attain mastery of life force energy for their self-defense and healing. Qigong continues to be a remarkably effective life force energy practice for millions of people worldwide.

The WHD teaches you how to perform diagnostic qigong exercises to help you pinpoint those organ systems that are most out of balance and sabotaging calorie-burning potential. The book goes on to show how to perform qigong exercises to balance those glands and organs most in need, thus enabling you to maintain a more efficient metabolism in the long term.

Before going on to transform your dieting experience by detailing these remarkable difference-making energy therapies, we must first uncover the real root of the problem by getting right to the heart of the matter.

CHAPTER 2

THE HEART OF THE MATTER

The Energy of Emotion

According to recent electrocardiogram research, the heart's electromagnetic field generates five times more energy than the brain's, and the amplitude of the heart's electrical field is sixty times greater than that of the brain. This is largely due to the powerful energy emitted by human emotion. We must remember that emotions are energy. We've known for years that the emotional energies of the heart are capable of producing dis-ease, but now science is beginning to learn that the emotional energies of the human heart also have the ability to balance and heal body, mind, and spirit. Researchers have discovered that the heart's electromagnetic field has a coding system that can transmit entrainment frequencies, generated by positive emotions, to assist with our rebalancing and reorganization following trauma or a stressful ordeal.

Each emotion produces a uniquely different electromagnetic frequency.

Positive emotions generate higher frequencies; negative emotions, lower frequencies. Higher emotional frequencies connote creative power, while negative emotional frequencies evince destructive force. The greater our tendency to harbor negative emotions, the lower our vibrational frequency, and the more likely we are to succumb to unhealthy and/or destructive behaviors. The more positive our emotional state and the higher our vibrational frequency, the more likely we are to cultivate healthy, creative behaviors. Everything is energy. Our emotional energies are powerful and forceful—so much so that they are often the root causes of our dis-ease.

Between 1995 and 2002 researcher and author Dr. David Hawkins calibrated the energy of specific human states of consciousness (including emotions) on a relative range from 0 to 1,000, with 0 representing the lowest and 1,000 the highest energy. He did this with the help of applied kinesiology. Again, the lower calibrations represent frequencies that contribute to dis-ease, and the higher calibrations generate states of ease. In his book *Power vs. Force*, Hawkins recorded the following calibrations, representing the three human emotions that generate the lowest frequencies:[1]

1. Shame: 20
2. Guilt: 30
3. Apathy: 50

The following calibrations from Hawkins represent the three human emotions that generate the highest frequencies:

1. Enlightenment: 700–1,000
2. Peace: 600
3. Joy: 540

Hawkins's energy calibrations inspired me to run some similar tests of my own. With the thought in mind that emotional forces lie at the causal root of our overeating, I was intrigued by the idea of performing some of my own kinesiology testing, in order to determine the three lowest-calibrating human emotions at the heart of the present weight gain and obesity problem. While clearly understanding that there are always a myriad of emotions at play here, I was resolute to discover the three principal emotional afflictions that cause us to overeat.

I did indeed decipher these emotional frequency calibrations with the help of my EMT system of kinesiology. For our purposes, kinesiology is the manual strength testing of the body's neuromuscular mechanics. It is a means for establishing the mind/body's positive or negative reaction to things like foods and nutritional supplements (for more on this, see chapter 6). Here's what I found.

The Three Emotional Overeating Frequencies
1. Fear—negative—relative 1,000 (1.1 Hz)
2. Shame—negative—relative 850 (1.4 Hz)
3. Apathy—negative—relative 770 (1.1 Hz)

On a more technical note, posted right beside each relative kinesiology calibration I've listed the exact frequency of each of the three principal overeating emotions in cycles per second, or hertz. It's these three main emotionally generated low frequencies that keep us from breaking old destructive eating patterns. If we're to overcome our struggle with food and chronic overeating we must first commit to contending with these three destructive emotional frequencies that take root deep within our hearts. It's time we realized that our struggle with weight gain and obesity is less about the food on our plate and more about the emotional energy in our hearts. It's not about fad dieting, but about getting to the heart of our fear, shame, and apathy.

Fear

One of the world's great models of energy healing, classical Chinese medicine, is based on a cosmological five element system, in which all within and everything between heaven and earth are constitutionally categorized into five metaphorical classifications: wood, fire, earth, metal, and water.

The five-element system tells us that fear is an emotion that resides within the kidneys, and joy is the emotion that resides within the heart. The kidneys symbolically represent the water element. The heart represents the fire element. The kidneys (water) are in charge of regulating the heart (fire). It is considered of vital importance for our water (fear) to regulate our fire (joy). For the same fire that can warm, cook, and shed light on our visions can also destroy everything. This offers an interesting and enlightening perspective, as it presents us with an image of fear as the principal governing force over our life's greatest potentials. When properly balanced, fear puts us in position to experience balanced joy. However, when our fear (water) is deficient, life's temptations are free to fan the flames of our destructive emotional fire. This is when mania, foolhardy confidence, and distorted risk taking result. The five-element wisdom tells us it's all about having a holistic appreciation of our fear.

Fear is generally thought of as an emotion induced by threats that are both real and/or perceived. Fear alters chemistry, brain, and organ function and behavior. If imbalanced, fear can have a paralyzing effect on the body, mind, and spirit. The single greatest obstacle that stands in the way of our healing and transformation is fear. Our most primal fear is our fear of pain. Our fear of pain comes in a myriad of forms: fear of feeling, fear of failure, fear of success, fear of loss, fear of shame, fear of guilt, etc. It's the fear of pain that most often keeps prospective dieters from ever getting started.

We have a growing population of overweight and obese people who desperately want to succeed at permanent weight loss, but they are so afraid of having to face the truth that they continue to buy into "the lie."

Afraid of the Truth

Listen closely to what I'm about to say. The first step in overcoming your chronic overweight and obesity problem is to stop being afraid of the truth! It's time you got to the heart of the matter!

Some of us are food addicts. Some of us are compulsive overeaters. Some of us are binge eaters. Some of us are stress eaters, and some of us are just overindulgers. Seventy-five percent of us overeat not because we're hungry but because of emotional pain.

For many of us, food has become a coping mechanism. Food can temporarily calm our nerves and distract us from painful emotions. It is arguably the quickest way for us to shift from negative to positive emotional energy frequencies. Unfortunately this solution is part of a problematic, vicious cycle that comes full circle from pain to pleasure and right back to pain again.

This cycle begins with destructive negative emotional frequencies generated from fear, shame, and apathy and culminates in obsessive overeating. Overeating means gaining weight. Gaining weight means we're right back to the fear, shame, and apathy. So, as we go deeper, we begin to realize that overeating is prompted by these negative emotions that set off a chronic destructive cycle.

There persists the stereotypical belief that overeating is simply due to a lack of willpower. Nothing could be further from the truth. When you go to the heart of the matter, you'll find that overeating is entwined with emotion, biochemistry, and neurology.

Emotional pain rooted in fear, shame, and apathy becomes embedded in the psyche, resulting in chronic depression, anxiety, and dissociation. The heavy burden imposed by these powerful negative emotional frequencies alters biochemistry to program the nervous system for addiction. The end result of this programming is lower levels of "feel-good" neurotransmitters like melatonin and serotonin, and elevated levels of cortisol.

Once this systemic emotional, biochemical, neurological connection gets traction, food will have an entirely different effect on the brain and body. The brain and body will have become accustomed to having their biochemical fires of stress put out by floods of endorphins, triggered by favorite foods. Now endogenous neuropeptides such as endorphins and enkephalins will have started binding to morphine-like receptors in the brain, turning food into a virtual opiate. The destructive cycle that results in overeating begins with emotions like fear. Therefore, the only way for us to break the cycle is to go deeper into the nature of our fear.

As a culture, we tend not to like getting our hands too dirty, especially regarding matters of the heart. We're a society weaned on heavenly pleasure and hell-bent on denying pain. We're just not inclined to go deep. We don't want to face the truth, but only by doing so will we be able to transcend the destructive frequencies of the fear that binds us.

As a young practitioner I was very much afraid of having to get to the heart of the matter with patients. Over time, however, I gradually developed a better comfort level. In fact, I discovered that taking such a risk was necessary to helping patients break through to a more effective level of healing. I will forever recall my first such risk-taking breakthrough.

A middle-aged gentleman who was an air traffic controller had come to see me in hopes of losing weight. He suffered from chronic anxiety and insomnia and had a history of struggling with addictions to tobacco, caffeine, and rich food. He was approximately fifty pounds overweight at the time. It was with great angst that he went on to explain how he'd spent most of his adult life as a failed fad dieter. He was clearly very discouraged about it, but I didn't get the sense that he was ready to throw in the towel. In fact, I could feel that he'd managed to maintain a strong commitment to his health. Anyone could plainly see that he was an intensely passionate man whose emotional energies ran deep—the fact that he wore his heart on his sleeve struck a chord with me.

At once, we unexpectedly found ourselves enwrapped in an intensely candid heart-to-heart communion. He wasted little time getting right to the root of his heart's discontent. Time seemed to stand still. It was as if our conversation was suddenly being channeled by forces greater than us. A fluid stream of consciousness flowed between us and he went on to divulge sensitive information about his painful childhood. It was without hesitation that he shared with me many of his most agonizing lifelong emotional frustrations. We were able to tap into some of the deepest causal roots tied to his chronic anxiety, insomnia, and addiction. This seemed to inspire the sparking of a positive, high-frequency emotion called hope. From that point on I could sense a dramatic energy shift in the man. We followed up with hourly office visits on a monthly basis, and upon completion of our six-month follow-up, he had attained his fifty-pound weight loss goal, and so much more.

Today he remains healthy, fit, and smoke-free. During our initial time together, we learned that food addiction and chronic weight gain are symptoms more than they are diseases, and that healing them demands a risk-taking willingness to rechannel the destructive emotional frequencies of the heart. The roots of every overeating problem trace back to the wounded heart of an inner child. Fear, shame, and apathy germinate within the subterranean soil of our fertile psyche very early on.

As Lisa Firestone put it in *Psychology Today*, "As children, we all experience varying degrees of emotional pain. The love, care, and nurturance we get from our caregivers lead us to form a positive sense of self and help us to create our identity. Yet, no parent or person is perfect. Even the best parents are only attuned to their child's needs about 30 percent of the time. This means that, as children, each of us was inevitably left lacking certain things we needed. We may have felt rejected, isolated, unseen, or unheard. Conversely, we may have felt intruded on, overly controlled, or intimidated by our parents. All of these factors could have impacted our relationship with food. We literally and figuratively learned how to 'feed' ourselves from how we were nurtured by our parents and influential caretakers."[2]

The fear, shame, and apathy that many of us experience as children often trigger distorted perceptions and dysfunctional, overcompensating behaviors. I've counseled many obese patients over the years who've openly confessed that they perceive their excess weight as a kind of armor protecting them from the frightening prospect of any further emotional pain. For them, food has become a protective shield. For many, food allays fear. The human mind can devise an infinite number of strategies to use food as a bulwark against fear.

A number of years ago I saw a woman in her midthirties who was a hundred pounds overweight. When I first took her diet history, I was surprised to discover that her food-based calorie intake was relatively balanced. However, her caloric intake of beverages was astronomically high. She was drinking liter upon liter of soda, juice, sugary drinks, and milk shakes. During the course of our meetings she told me that she was an only child who was raised by a single mother. She said that her mother was just too stressed and overwhelmed to provide the nurturance she so desperately needed. She recalled often being completely ignored while lying in her crib crying for her bottle. She said that as she evolved into her teenage years she started to feel increasingly driven to consume as many liquid calories as she possibly could to compensate for the deprivation and pain of her childhood.

Food has forever been used as a remedy to compensate for our crippling fear of the truth. It's the pacifying milk from a mother's breast, it's the comforting ice cream after skinning our knee, it's the lollipop after learning that our best childhood friend has to move away. Our codependent relationship with food extends from the depths of our heart and soul to our brain and nervous system, resulting in a dis-ease that manifests as destructive, obsessive, and addictive behaviors. In order for us to heal ourselves of this systemic dis-ease process we must overcome our fear of the truth.

Fear and Denial

Everything is energy. All the energy in the cosmos is dynamic, variable, and in a constant state of flux. All forms of energy respond to the animating push of flux with either flow or resistance. In other words, change is constant. We can choose to go with it, or we can resist it. When we go with the forces of change, the result is energetic flow. When we resist change, the result is tension. The greater our resistance to change, the greater the tension we must contend with.

Denial is resistance—resistance to truth. The longer we insist on denying the truth, the greater the degree of tension we'll be forced to contend with. If the truth is that chronic overweight and obesity problems are rooted in eating dysfunction, and eating dysfunction is rooted in emotional pain from fear, shame, and apathy, then the only logical conclusion one could arrive at is that fad dieting is a form of denial—denial of emotional pain.

Perhaps the greatest of all human temptations is to deny emotional pain. That is, until one day we come to realize that emotional pain is undeniable. To deny pain is to welcome suffering. A Buddhist friend of mine once put this in perspective. He explained that to believe that we have a choice between pleasure and pain is but an illusion. He went on to share the Buddhist perspective that the only real choice we truly have is between short-term pain and long-term suffering. He noted that short-term pain is more intense, but that a willingness to face it head-on allows us to move more swiftly through its process, and on to liberation. He then pointed out that long-term suffering is the natural result of denial. When we attempt to deny our short-term pain, our suffering only becomes more unrelenting—instead of liberation, we become afflicted by pain's bondage. Denial, with its resultant suffering, is a state to which far too many of us remain forever fastened.

A brief examination of our use of language reveals our reluctance to face our pain head-on. The energy has been virtually drained out of some of our most powerful words—all to suit our inclination to live in denial. The word "stress" is arguably the most commonly used word we choose to describe pain. In fact, it's become one of the most frequently used words in our vocabulary. There's little doubt that a word like "stress" should indeed have a striking impact. Yet, strangely enough, its greatest power now lies not in what it says, but rather in what it fails to say.

The word "stress" has essentially been neutered in order to keep us from having to acknowledge what's really going on emotionally within us. It has virtually lost all of its meaning. It's merely become a part of our colloquial lexicon—an insignificant conversation filler.

In point of fact, "stress" actually refers to a cascade of disorienting chemical changes that become activated in the body whenever strong emotional energies get gridlocked. Repressed emotions are what produce the energy that triggers the plethora of symptoms most commonly associated with physiological stress.

Denial then activates the brain, mind, and nervous system, further actuating the release of hormones like cortisol, which increases sugar cravings, and aldosterone, which drives up salt cravings. Acute and chronic stress dramatically increases levels of these two hormones, ultimately resulting in a cycle of sugar cravings followed by salt cravings. Once this cycle is biochemically bolstered, there are only two ways for us to respond—to feed the food down or to feel the emotions out.

This brings us full circle, right back to the concept of flow versus resistance. By denying the powerful emotional frequencies within us, we're choosing to resist the physics of our own power and force. By saying no to the flow of emotional energy that's demanding to move through us, we're accumulating frustrated tension that can only result in dis-ease. The tension that builds from such denial then progresses from failed dieting frustration to failed serial dieting frustration to an intensification of food addiction. The more we deny the pain, the more it suppurates. The greater our pain, the stronger becomes our drive to make the hurting stop.

Fear of Being Without the Comforting Love of Food

A little over two million years ago, our ancestors first began hunting big game. Big game like woolly mammoths couldn't be hunted and killed by small tribes and cave clans—thus, hunting and eating became social events. Around that same time, the human brain was in its early stages of formulating the hippocampal hormones—leptin and ghrelin—vital to memory and emotional development, as well as dopamine, which regulates the brain's reward centers. Let's just say that as of two million years ago we humans no longer needed to be reminded whom we'd enjoyed our most recent dining pleasures with. We ate in groups, shared in the pleasures with friends and neighbors, and developed fond memories around the experience. Just as true today as it was then, our brains associate food with memory-making emotions.

Today we celebrate virtually every aspect of life together with food. We make love with food, we celebrate life with food, and we memorialize our losses with food. We've always had an abiding relationship with food—a relationship that reaches deep into the innermost recesses of our soul. Life is complicated and demanding, and through all the changes, challenges, and heartaches, food has always been there with us, and for us. Our lives and lifestyles have forever been associated with food, feelings, and memories.

The human mind is a memory machine with an affinity for making associative connections. I recall stumbling upon an associative memory study of people who'd suffered abuse. The study was able to consistently show biofeedback spikes in vital functions whenever the subjects viewed colors that were associated with the colors of their perpetrators' clothing, some twenty to thirty years after the fact. This study supports the theory that, subconsciously, we never forget.

For most of us, food has found a way into our hearts and associatively linked itself to some of our most impressionable memories. As you're reading this page, I'm certain that you can recall both old and recent memories that you've unconsciously associated with food, like a holiday dinner with family and friends or an intimate, romantic candlelight dinner with someone special. There's no question about it—for most of us, the thought of food elicits powerful emotional memories.

One study, performed by associate professor of nutrition David Vanata of Ashland University in Ohio, found that by merely thinking about various foods, subjects expressed varying degrees of happiness, excitability, pleasantness, and comfort. As you might imagine, the highest happiness scores went to ice cream, chocolate, cake, grapes, and pizza. Overall, the highest-ranking foods for emotional response when combining happiness, excitability, pleasantness, and comfort scores turned out to be ice cream, chocolate, and cookies.[3] Our experience with food is emotionally associative. Associative memories elicit powerful emotions, and powerful emotions engage sensory neurology linking the emotions and memories to sights, sounds, smells, feelings, and tastes.

Science is discovering powerful links between our sensory connections with food and our early life experiences. Similar to the way we as adults might associate the fragrance of a certain perfume or cologne with a lover, we create strong sensory bonds between food and the pleasant memories in our life.

For me, the fragrance of a rich tomato sauce immediately stirs fond memories of cooking and dining with my beautiful Italian grandmother, Maria Nina De La Fabiano. I spent a good deal of my childhood enjoying her love and the warmth of her surroundings. I shall never forget assisting her with the culinary creation of a soup she referred to as *minestra*. Once a week she'd take just about everything in her refrigerator that was on the verge of being thrown out and put it in a large soup pot of boiling water and spices. Upon completion of her minestra masterpiece, we'd sit together and enjoy sharing in the love and laughter as we partook of a bowl of "you name it" soup together. This memory-making would often carry over to the next morning. Whenever I was fortunate enough to spend the night at Grandma's, I'd often awaken to a breakfast of Cheerios swimming in a bowl of coffee, cream, and sugar. And though I don't drink coffee today, I do often find myself inhaling its ambrosial scent, and each time I do, I return to the same special memory. Like most of us, I have many happy, loving memories around food. I do have some not-so-happy memories around food that remain with me as well.

I recall an occasion when I was a young boy and my mother asked me if I'd like to have hot dogs and beans for lunch. Excitedly, I answered, "Yes, please!" Moments later I found myself staring at a plate of lima beans. I know it's not unusual for a mom to occasionally pull a fast one in an attempt to sneak in a new food from time to time, but this was one of those times I was simply having none of it. I distinctly recall digging my heels in, determined not to eat these disgusting little green earlobe-shaped things. Unfortunately for me, Mom had her game face on that day. Our wills were poised and a battle royal ensued, and I was not allowed to leave that table for what seemed like an eternity. To this day, I've never eaten a lima bean, and I never will! In fact, the mere mention of them instantly ushers me back in time to that distressing moment in my life.

We've all made powerful associative connections between food, emotion, and neurology that reveal our deep, abiding relationship with food. Food has been our only friend in the world, and food has been our worst enemy. Food has been our poison and our miracle cure, and it has often both caused and eased our pain.

There's been a good deal of research that's shown that at least some of the effects of food on our mood trace back to our primitive biology. One series of recent studies discovered that subjects who had full stomachs while listening to sad music and looking at sad faces experienced positive mood shifts. Researchers say that it points to evolutionary programming that was designed to keep us alive when food was scarce. The authors of these studies theorize that due to the fact that this primitive chemistry has become obsolete, it's now likely contributing mightily to our current obesity problem.

Other studies have found that high stress drives up emotional eating by triggering powerful glucocorticoid receptors in the taste buds that stimulate our desire for starchy, sugary, fatty comfort foods. Studies such as these have made it clear that when you combine our current easy access to food with our primitive survival chemistry, the result is uncontrollable eating. Throw in exceedingly high levels of emotional stress and you've got yourself an obesity dilemma. Our history, memories, survival chemistry, and high levels of stress all contribute to our powerful emotional connection to food. Our relationship with food runs deep.

Shame

As we all know, nothing can ever fill any void left by the absence of real love. Nonetheless, our growing addiction to food is one surefire indicator that real love is waning in our world. The world will never overcome addiction without replacing its self-contempt with self-love.

Why do we suffer from such self-contempt? In a word, the answer is shame. Ours has become an increasingly competitive cultural experiment. We compete in the home. We compete in the classroom and schoolyard. Many of us go on to compete in college and at our jobs. The results are always the same—more failure than success. When you get right down to it, it's really not so much about our successes or failures. It's more about the feelings we've been programmed to attach to them. We learn very early on to link negative emotional energies like fear to the prospect of success, and likewise to link shame to failure.

I recently had a session with a thirty-five-year-old woman who suffers from chronic stress and anxiety. She nervously entered my office, in a state of great angst. I asked why she was so nervous and advised her to distill her overwhelming feelings down to their causal root. She said she was anxious and afraid of being late for our appointment. I once again suggested that we distill things a bit more, so I asked her what she thought would happen if she were to arrive late for our appointment. She said that by arriving late and/or missing out on our appointment, she felt she might lose both the fee and the opportunity for treatment, which would have been interpreted as a shameful failure on her behalf. We talked further and she went on to explain that her mother had had an extremely critical nature and had always shamed her and made her feel inadequate when she was growing up. She told me that she'd always wanted to be a lawyer or a teacher, but that her mother demanded instead that she attend secretarial school. She said that her mother programmed her not to fail. Subsequently, she recalled struggling with anxiety, fear of failure, and shame most of her life.

I inquired as to what, if any, collateral damage she believed this may have caused her. She said that she thought the stress from a lifetime of shame affected her overall emotional state, heart rate, blood pressure, and immune system. She told me that, looking back on it, she was quite certain that her mother suffered from OCD, which she believed her mother had developed from the shame and stress of being an abandoned, motherless child.

I asked her to close her eyes for a moment, take a few deep breaths, and imagine that she was viewing a past mother-daughter episode from the movie of her life. I suggested that she visualize her present-day adult self stepping into this scene from her past so that she might bring some healing to the situation. I asked her what she'd like to tell the spirit of her mother and her "child self" if she could. She said that she'd like to tell them, "Stop trying so hard! There's no need to be perfect! You're both fine just the way you are! Enjoy life! Take the time to have more fun and enjoy each other!" Tears began to well up in her eyes as she reflected on her many years of suffering from toxic shame.

"Toxic shame, the shame that binds you, is experienced as the all-pervasive sense that 'I'm flawed and defective as a human being,'" writes John Bradshaw in *Healing the Shame That Binds You*. "Toxic shame is no longer an emotion—it signals our limits. It's a state of being—a core identity. Toxic shame gives you a sense of worthlessness, a sense of failing and falling short as a human being. Toxic shame is a rupture of the self with the self.

"Toxic shame is so excruciating because it is the painful exposure of the believed failure of self to the self. In toxic shame, the self becomes an object of its own content, an object that can't be trusted. As an object that can't be trusted, one experiences oneself as untrustworthy. Toxic shame is experienced as an inner torment, a sickness of the soul. If I'm an object that can't be trusted, then I'm not in me. Toxic shame is paradoxical and self-generating."[4]

The stress and depletion that result from this self-generating emotion trigger a cycle of dis-ease.

I recently visited with a patient whom I see once a year, usually during the summer. She suffers from chronic, seasonal mononucleosis and binge eating, brought on by very busy, stressful spring and summer work overloads. She's relatively symptom free in the winter months, when her business slows down. She explained that her cyclical symptoms are triggered by a lifetime of stress, which she traces back to workaholic programming downloaded into her by her father when she was a kid. Dad was a workaholic, and so his daughter has been unconsciously programmed to not become a "shameful slacker"—so much so, it's caused a cyclical pattern of chronic immunosuppression and obsessive-compulsive binge eating in her life.

I recommended an antiviral diet with some immune-enhancing nutritional supplements, but for at least twenty of the thirty minutes that we worked together, I encouraged her to consciously work at uprooting her dis-ease by breaking her shame-based thought patterns. The specific dysfunctional messages that she most needs to uproot are that slackers are not deserving of their own love, and that unless she's willing to work herself sick, she should see herself as nothing but a shameful slacker.

Repeated shaming ultimately distorts self-image to a point of chronic self-contempt, and chronic self-contempt inevitably leads to destructive behaviors. "The world's constant rejection has at last convinced me that I'm flawed. Now I'm beginning to resent myself for being so unattractive to a world that I so desperately need. Therefore, I'm left no other alternative than to agree with the world. I don't like me either. In fact, I don't like me so much that I just might destroy this flawed, unattractive self once and for all."

I have a very dear friend of many years who was one of the most remarkable and gifted men ever to walk the earth. Unfortunately, he was the last to know it. In fact, he never got it, which is why he's no longer with us. When I first met him he was a tobacco-, alcohol-, and drug-addicted teenager. He eventually got clean and sober, but then decided to turn his addiction to food. He gained eighty-five pounds in a relatively short period of time, and then I got ahold of him. He followed the nutritional program I designed for him and he eventually got down to a healthy weight again. He seemed to be getting himself back on track. He was divinely blessed with extraordinary gifts and talents. He had a beautiful and loving wife, four magnificent children, and many deeply devoted friends, but there always seemed to be something missing. No matter how good his life was, he was unable to enjoy the ride.

His father was an austere, critical figure who found it difficult to play an intimate, unconditionally loving role in his son's life. It was clear to many who knew him that the absence of his father's love left a fathomless void. Moreover, it resulted in a critical inner voice that tormented him right up until the end. Thousands showered him with love during his last days, but all the love in the world couldn't heal him from the bottomless pain of his deep-seated shame and self-contempt.

Shame and Self-Abandonment

The word "addiction" comes from the Latin *addicere*, meaning "to enslave." As long as we're devoid of self-love, we'll remain vulnerable to the torment of our own critical voices within. It's these shaming voices of self-destruction that prevail upon us to stuff ourselves full of anything other than self.

We Americans account for approximately 4.6 percent of the global population, yet we consume 80 percent of the world's opiates. The fact that our opiate use continues to skyrocket at such an alarming rate is a clear sign that our pain is insurmountable. In fact, you might say that our pain is surpassed only by our determination to not feel it. In parts of the major population centers of the United States, oxycodone-based products such as OxyContin, Percocet, and Percodan are said to have increased sixteenfold over the past decade. There is a great void within that we're fruitlessly attempting to fill with substances like these.

In 1943, noted American psychologist Abraham Maslow published "A Theory of Human Motivation," in *Psychological Review*. The gist of his message was that in order to be a truly fulfilled human being, one must have a hierarchy of five vital needs met. Here's one interpretation of what Maslow's hierarchy might look like:

1. Self-actualization (performance talent, creativity, and fulfillment)
2. Self-esteem (achievement, mastery, and recognition)
3. Belonging (friends, family, and community)
4. Safety (security and protection from danger)
5. Basic physiological needs (food, water, and warmth)

The most important takeaway stems from the first two, Maslow's "self-actualization" and "self-esteem": Without self-love, it's virtually impossible for our core to be fulfilled. In the absence of self-love, there can be no love at all. With no vital connection to our indwelling life spring, we are left to operate our lives out of a void. Maslow tells us that if we are to prosper, this void must be filled by self, with self. When there is no self through which to live life, a primal instinct to belong to something else rises up as a force of desperation from within. When we're not "self" connected, we're destined to become "other" connected—we simply cannot survive being disconnected. But in a world where "the real thing" is so hard to come by, chances are better than good that "other" will not be there to love our "self," because "other" will be preoccupied with its own struggle to find fulfillment. After we've been repeatedly turned away, desperation soon follows. The more desperate we become, the more likely we are to broaden our fulfillment search.

It doesn't take a human being very much rejection for him or her to be drawn to the myriad of pleasure-providing options that are available. Of all those options, food is arguably the most accessible form of instant gratification. Food has long been the object of our desire for its mere ability to instantly fill us full. It comes right down to *feeling* or *feeding*.

Experts tell us that most of our overeating is caused by recurring negative emotional states. These emotional states have the power to rewire our brains and nervous systems, creating an unquenchable physiological desire for food. Our bad moods dramatically increase our desire for foods that satisfy defective insulin receptors. Thus, chronic negative emotions can set up vicious cycles of addictive overeating. If you break the human heart enough times, the emotional repercussions ultimately alter body-mind and brain chemistries. There are powerful opiate centers in the brain that produce neurotransmitters like dopamine, serotonin, and endorphins that offset negative emotions. This chemistry results in a neurology that reinforces emotion and results in chronic compulsive behavior. Make no mistake about it: food has the power to possess our body, mind, and spirit.

Many years ago, I was asked to give a presentation at an aestheticians' conference in Wellesley, Massachusetts. About ten minutes before I was to begin my talk, the spirit moved me to jot down the following words on a piece of paper: "Complete the following sentence by filling in the blank: Food is _____." Approximately two hundred people were in attendance that evening, so I asked the organizers if there was a nearby copying machine that I might use. I quickly proceeded to run off a few hundred copies, then asked for assistance placing them on all the chairs in the room moments before beginning. As the attendees filed into the room and took their seats, they were asked to fill in the blank on the page. After a few minutes their responses were collected, and as I read them I was immediately taken aback by what I saw. This group, mostly very attractive, fit, well-dressed, educated women, opened my eyes to something that night that I never forgot. Here are some of the answers that appeared:

Food is—Love.
Food is—Life.
Food is—Death.
Food is—Heartache.
Food is—Pain and suffering.
Food is—Hopelessness.

It was clear to me that many of the people in that room that night were feeling pretty empty. Food had clearly become far too important to them in all the wrong ways. But a quick examination of their answers tells us that food isn't the real problem. It's the systematic disempowerment and abandonment of "self."

For food has clearly been bequeathed unlimited "other" power. Look at how much power many of these women assigned to food. A good number of them answered that food is love. What really comes through loud and clear here is the self-abandonment that manifests as a lack of self-love. We're simply not raised to fully occupy and love "self." So here we are. Most of us don't even know what it means to love ourselves. Meanwhile, no one wants to be lonely and feel unloved—so enter the "other," otherwise known as food. But food is not the answer. Food temporarily fills the emptiness, but it cannot fulfill the void. The more deprived of true fulfillment one is, the more addicted to the notion of being filled full one becomes.

If you were to distill compulsive and addictive behavior down to its causal roots, you'd find shame and self-abandonment. Shame and self-abandonment trigger the insidious pathology of food's potentially life-damaging, mood-altering force. Painful, flawed perceptions of self drive the biology of addiction. What starts out as distorted emotion and thought ultimately transmutes into neurological and biochemical addiction. It's all about turning off the "pain" switch.

Food makes us feel better without having to wait. Biochemically, this gratification response gains immediate access to our brain's reward center (nucleus accumbens). The nervous system is the first to feel the "feel-good" endorphin reaction of this instant gratification response. In short, we go from feeling really bad to feeling really good in milliseconds. As Mara Tyler reports on healthline .com, "Research, such as a 2010 study published in *Current Opinion in Gastroenterology*, shows increasing evidence that food addiction is a result of changes in a person's neurochemistry and neuroanatomy. . . . When lab rats were given free access to high-fat, high-sugar foods, their brains changed. The changes in their behavior and physiology were similar to the changes caused by drug abuse."[5] Study after study reveals that the biochemical changes imposed by foods are instantaneous, powerful, and lasting. This is the reason their chemical reactions are tied to a lifetime of emotion.

The indelible pain from a lifetime of internalized shame makes us feel chronically depressed and anxious, but it doesn't take long for our brains and nervous systems to discover that food can soothe that pain in no time at all.

Shame and self-abandonment produce a quaking in the heart that only fulfillment can ease. Without love, food becomes an available proxy. But like any surrogate love, this fix doesn't last for very long. Food's endorphin response is only good until the next mouthful. Before long, deprived endorphin receptors begin sending powerful craving signals to our nervous systems: "We're starting to feel the hurt again. We're getting jittery. We need more." Thus, the addiction process has been biochemically effectuated. That which was once distorted emotions and thoughts has at last become encoded into our neurochemistry. The damaging, state-altering potential of this destructive cycle from shame to self-abandonment to addiction is noxious.

Feeling Instead of Feeding

Anita N. was a bright, affable, fifty-two-year-old woman who reported in at five feet, six inches and 320 pounds. She had struggled unsuccessfully with five or six diet programs in the past and decided to give a personalized, one-on-one approach a try. We immediately rolled up our sleeves and got started by kinesiologically testing her foods and setting a nutritional plan. She seemed to get good traction right off the bat, as each of her first successive follow-ups revealed excellent results. Anita's father had died when she was much younger—and, subsequently, she and her mother were still living together. It wasn't too long before I had the opportunity to meet her mother and observe their relationship dynamics. I could see right away that there was a great deal of tension between the two. Her mother was very critical of her, especially her weight problem and eating habits. She would often betray Anita's confidence by calling me to tell me she'd discovered fast food wrappers under Anita's bed and in her drawers and closets. Eventually, I had to stop taking her phone calls, as she insisted on ignoring my coaching input. Her mother's critical nature and shaming tactics stirred self-contempt and anger in Anita. The dysfunctional tension between the two clearly stirred up a rebellious streak in Anita, which ended up sabotaging her good intentions.

A clear cyclical pattern began to avail itself. Periods of exceptional results by Anita were followed by spells of anger at her mother and shame about herself, followed by periods of weight gain. It was time for Anita and me to have a good talk. I made it clear straightaway that her frustrating relationship with her mother was setting her off on emotional eating binges. Without hesitation, she affirmed my assertion and began to cry. She clearly understood that her conflict of loving her mother but being very angry with and shamed by her left her feeling uncontrollable anger. She explained that these conflicting emotions made her feel trapped in her own body. She told me that she loved her mother far too much to contend with the degree of anger that she felt. Thus, her conscious mind had turned the problem over to her unconscious mind, which decided to stuff down with food the energy of her frustration, shame, and anger.

Anita was now conscious of the fact that she was an emotional eater. I told her that with all emotional eaters, it comes down to the decision to "feed" or "feel." I explained to her that emotions are very powerful energies and that feeding represents "energy in" and feeling represents "energy out." I advised her to be mindful of her feelings. I told her that anytime they came up, she'd best bear responsibility for releasing their potentially dis-ease–producing energy. I explained that by feeling instead of feeding, she'd be able to overcome her emotional toxicity and at last be free to embrace her dark side.

Healing Our Shame: Embracing Our Dark Side

Like everything in the universe, we are composed of both energy and matter. Similarly, we are composed of a lower human nature and a higher spirit nature. Our lower human nature is easy to identify with. It's the carnal, fallible part of us that is chronically plagued by temptation, confusion, and emotional pain. Our higher spirit nature, on the other hand, is that transcendent part of us that has the power to protect, inspire, and uplift us. It's our supernatural overdrive for those times when we're stuck on life's highway. Our higher spirit nature is the "get real" part of us that reveals itself on the rarest of occasions. Our collective higher spirit was very much in evidence during and after September 11, 2001. It was as if we'd mystically undergone a transformational unification during those shocking days.

While it's easy to interpret our higher spirit nature as good and our lower human nature as less than good, it's important to remember that together, these two divergent representations of self make up our wholeness. It is due to the fact that our lower human nature is correlated with the darkness of temptation, confusion, and emotional pain that we're inclined to identify it as evil. The evil, however, comes not from our lower human nature, but from the world's influence over it.

Each of these components of self is plugged into a different energy source. Our lower human nature is attuned to the energy of the world. Our higher spirit nature is tuned into the innate stream of consciousness that flows from deep within and all around us. It's as though we have two different selves that are unconsciously modulated by the frequencies of two entirely different programming networks. The frequencies of the world so distort our vulnerable human nature that most of us end up unconsciously blaming and ultimately loathing ourselves for our mortal iniquities.

It's important to remember that we are human beings with two distinctly different selves. The presence of one naturally falls away as the other rises. It's essential that we remain ever aware of the addictive influences around us at all times—it's also important to forgive our lower human selves for their natural attraction to those influences. Self-solidarity is the only antidote for personal shame, but integral wholeness is a choice that demands ever-present awareness. It all begins with living moment to moment in a state of conscious attunement, fully aware of what energy network our thoughts are tuned into.

What frequency is your mind harmonized with? What's the general theme of your internal narrative? What's the spirit of your inner dialogue? Are you attuned to the voice of the world, or are you tapped into the universal stream of consciousness? The world network's signals can get very staticky, to say the least. Are you aware of your awareness enough to be able to change the station in your mind to a higher frequency when need be? Can you get yourself unstuck from the lower-frequency dial? Does the network you're tuned to remind you that half of your self is naturally created of darkness, and that the collective darkness of the world is continually attempting to manipulate it?

I recently visited with a thirty-year-old mother of three who is a girls' lacrosse coach. She first came to see me determined to lose weight, and recently she came in excited to share the news that she'd lost over twenty pounds. Even more important, she was anxious to discuss some of the transformational changes that she'd been experiencing. She shared a story with me about how she'd unconsciously become entranced by her depressing, shaming, critical inner voice. She told me that the voice had come very close to destroying her life. Then one day, while looking at the lacrosse team pictures with a dear friend and fellow coach who also happened to be overweight, she couldn't help but notice that in virtually every photograph, her friend was pictured in the back, far behind everyone else. She asked her friend why she was in the back of every picture. Her friend told her that ever since she was a young child, whenever it was time for a group picture, she would always creep unsuspectingly behind everyone else to hide her body from view. When my client heard her friend's sad admission, a voice in her head spoke the words, "I'm not doing this anymore!" She told me that she made a decision that day to begin unconditionally accepting herself and to start celebrating her life.

I told her that she'd made a conscious decision to "change the station" and that it would be extremely important for her to continue paying attention to this new mind-set. Moreover, I reminded her to never stop unconditionally embracing her dark side. I told her that it was not her lower human nature that had been bringing her down all those years—it was the world's influence over it.

I've worked with many overweight and obese people over the years and can attest to the fact that most who made a conscious connection with their higher spirit while managing to unconditionally embrace their dark side were much better equipped to deal with the pain that leads to addictive eating.

Shame disintegrates all sense of oneness. It provokes the detestation and abandonment of self. Food fills the vacuum left by the abandonment of self, but without providing true, lasting fulfillment. The only stabilizing fulfillment that can ground us in the face of such enmity is self-love. Self-love is a quantum stretch for anyone inculcated by years of self-loathing. It's a little less of a stretch to approach this from the perspective of duality equaling wholeness. Here's what I mean: The simple logic of one plus one equaling two, and two being an even, whole number is a simple way to say that when conjoined, two polar opposites make up one complete whole.

There is a perfect metaphorical depiction of what I am trying to convey in the great tai chi circle (commonly referred to as the "yin/yang" symbol).

The great circle represents a paradoxical metaphor that invites us to delve deeper into the potential holism of our duality. It is composed of half darkness and half light, symbolizing the interdependency of our lower and higher selves. It serves as a symbolic reminder that in the absence of either our darkness or our light, there can be no wholeness. The great circle teaches us that by failing to embrace our lower self, our higher self is destined to remain un-whole. The supreme state of oneness can result only when the two extremes are integrated.

Transcending Our Shame: Trusting in Our Own Inner Light

Once we become attuned to the higher frequencies of our innate stream of consciousness we tend to become less "other" and more "self" directed. Therefore, we begin getting our problem-solving advice from a higher source. So, where do you get your problem-solving advice from? In your time of greatest need, who's your problem-solving expert?

Whenever we use the word "expert," we're generally talking about someone else, or some "other." Most of us are not accustomed to thinking of ourselves as experts. Even those who are experts in some field often find themselves referring to someone else as the expert, much if not most of the time. Knowledge isn't just power—it is the power that makes the expert the expert. So, when it comes to the power of expertise, most of us have been programmed to think of ourselves as buyers. In our culture, we're persuaded to believe that power is an entitlement of expertise, representative of "other," not "self."

From very early on in life we're programmed to believe that powers rest with some "other"—God, mother, father, big brother, teacher, or coach. Knowledge, wisdom, and command are synonymous with "other." Therefore, we're constantly reaching outward beyond the presupposed limitations of "self" in search of knowledge, love, and approval from "other."

I've had many thousands of consultations, over more than three decades, with people who've come to me in search of vital information. Much to their surprise, the most important information I share with them is information that encourages them to stop reaching out and to start reaching in. I make it very clear that their most meaningful answers flow forth from the innate stream within them.

How many times have you watched a sporting event only to see an athlete point up to the heavens as if some "supreme other" were sitting on a throne thirty thousand feet above them and presiding over their accomplishment? You can walk into virtually any place of worship at any given time and find people praying in an outward direction, as if the divinity they're appealing to were residing in some distant domain far removed from the wretched habitat of "self." "Other" is perceived as immortal, while "self" is seen as mortal.

We've been subtly indoctrinated to surrender our power of "self" to the forces of "other"—so much so that many of us are now afraid to trust in the power of our own light. Moreover, by disempowering "self," "self" becomes exceedingly vulnerable to the attraction and addiction to "other." As long as we remain entranced under the spell of "other" power, we shall remain susceptible to the allure of its false promises. Turn on your television or radio for five minutes and consciously observe the programming. It's all about the self-imposed pseudopower of "other" seeking to capitalize on the natural human vulnerabilities of "self." Our bodies aren't fit and firm enough. Our teeth aren't white enough. Our hair isn't thick enough. God forbid you're over fifty and happen to be watching a Touch of Gray or Viagra commercial. The pummeling our human nature takes from the world's voice is unceasing.

We all have access to an innate stream of light that emanates from our source.

As long as we're distracted by world static, we'll remain tuned out of source wisdom. The inner voice of source wisdom represents our only access to true transcendent power—the only power capable of breaking our addictive link to "other."

Apathy

I define apathy as feeling defeated and shamed past the point of caring. Just yesterday I had a conversation with a male patient in his thirties who first came to me after having been diagnosed with acute inflammatory colitis. He wasn't able to hold down any food at all and was sick, weak, and at a breaking point. Over the course of the next several months, however, his strict dietary discipline resulted in a complete recovery. He was at last able to digest his food healthfully. He told me that he recently tried to encourage an extremely overweight acquaintance to come see me for weight loss. He told me the person's reply was, "I could never follow a diet like you're on. I just don't have the strength and determination." Mind you, we're talking about a potentially life-threatening issue. Nonetheless, like so many others, this person likely feels defeated and shamed past the point of caring.

As previously mentioned, nobody wins all the time. In fact, in this world there's more losing than winning, and repeated losing leads to deepening feelings of shame and inadequacy. If we are continually made to feel inadequate, the shaming effect is likely to become embedded in our spirit. Once we're dispirited, the door to addiction starts to swing open a little wider.

Instead of providing real solutions for this crippling state, the material world prefers to offer costly, artificial solutions. Solutions that fail to provide long-term results tend to produce negative side effects and, worse, leave us constantly coming back for more.

Every culture is a social experiment designed to improve the quality of life for those who qualify. Our framework was designed to improve life quality by providing material comfort. The message of our free enterprise system has always been, "And to the victor go the spoils." The most aggressive, intelligent, and attractive among us are given the greatest access to the best quality of life. Our thirst for perfection is unquenchable, and our appetite for winning is insatiable.

Ours has become a highly pressurized cultural experiment, replete with loss, riddled with shame, and devoid of self-love. The higher we raise our standards, the greater the probability of loss and failure, and continual loss and failure give way to the fracturing of the spirit. You can't imagine how many perfectly fit patients I meet with who insist that I help them to lose fifteen pounds. Far worse still than the shame is the apathy. I continually hear overweight and obese patients utter words like, "I hate myself," "I feel like I'll never lose this weight," and "I'm getting so I just don't seem to care anymore."

Our struggle to survive in spite of our own degraded self-image becomes intense. You might say that shame forces us to care too much for our own good. After years of caring too much, we just get burned out. That's when the apathy and self-contempt set in.

A sixty-six-year-old woman recently came to see me suffering from acid reflux, bladder inflammation, insomnia, memory impairment, concentration problems, panic, anxiety, and depression. I performed EMT energy diagnosis on her, which revealed that her symptoms traced back to her adrenal medulla, indicating severe and chronic stress. It was clear that the roots of her disharmony ran deep. She conveyed a pattern of stress-borne dis-ease that resulted from a lifelong disconnection from positivity and self-love. Her long-suffering spirit had been so deprived of joy that apathy had begun to set in. Her drive to survive had burned her out. I then explained that only by reformatting her mind, from a consciousness of survival to a consciousness of abundance, might she be able to inch her way back to some semblance of self-love. That was when she broke down in tears and told me that both her parents were Holocaust survivors. As we talked further, it became clear that the morphic resonance (emotional absorption) she'd experienced from living with survival-scarred parents all those years had so embedded itself in her psyche that it prevented her from fully feeling love and prosperity. The release of tears and strong emotions preceded a profound healing breakthrough. Her apathy had been broken. In fact, her heart had revealed to her that it had cared all the while.

Healing Our Apathy with Our Words

The concept of holism reminds us that healing can be invoked in body, mind, or spirit, and that to heal any one of these is to heal them all. Because the spirit resides within the infinite domain of the human mind, it's an unequaled source of great healing power.

Neuroscience tells us that our unconscious mind can process hundreds of billions of bits of information per second. Unfortunately, a vast majority of those thoughts are unconscious and negative. It's been said that our negative thoughts are like Velcro and our positive thoughts are like Teflon. So we humans tend to be somewhat negative by nature, as our brains were wired that way for survival purposes. Mother Nature saw fit to make sure we expected the worst for our own good, but she also gave us the option to either remain in this negative survival mode or choose to rewire our brains for something more upbeat.

You see, our brains are not hardwired—they're "neuroplastic," or designed for change. The act of rewiring the brain begins with changing the mind, and changing the mind begins with changing our thoughts. The nouveau science of neuroplasticity has discovered that rewiring the human brain and nervous system from negative to positive is largely a matter of changing the inner dialogue from negative to positive. Words alone have the power to change brain chemistry. It's of the utmost importance that the positive inner dialogue be repeated with great frequency. Our apathy can be turned around with our words.

In the brain change programs that I've developed for both individual and corporate use, I've discovered that it's extremely important that the positive phrases, or mantras, that one chooses for one's brain reformatting be exaggerated. For example, rather than choosing a languid phrase like "I love life," one might better select a more ostentatious positive phrase, such as "I am the master of the universe." The reason for this is that it's important to command the attention of the nervous system. I always remind my neuroplasticity subjects that a transformational mantra doesn't have to be accurate or true. It does have to be positive and attention getting. A number of the group programs that I've run over the years have clearly demonstrated that if you repeat an attention-getting positive mantra like "I am the master of the universe" for four minutes, twice a day, over a period of sixteen weeks, the brain will neurologically rewire itself from right-prefrontal-dominant negativity to left-prefrontal-dominant positivity. We have the power to overcome our apathy with words. Words of power, frequently repeated, stimulate the brain to rewire the nervous system from a negative to a positive mind-set. If we're accustomed to living in a hellish place and we want out, we might consider mending our mind by reformatting our inner dialogue. By simply changing our inner dialogue, we can engage our inner power.

In the words of the author Emmet Fox in his classic *Find and Use Your Inner Power*, "Both heaven and hell are states of consciousness, the net resultant of our beliefs and feelings at any time. Formerly, people thought that both heaven and hell were places where one went after death, and nowadays many people seem to think that neither heaven nor hell exists at all. The truth is that both hell and heaven do exist, but they are states of mind, and we experience them right here on this earth now."[6]

When you have true peace of mind and an adequate understanding of life, you are already in heaven. When you are full of fear, anxiety, hatred, or physical pain, you are in hell. The conventional descriptions of both places are but an attempt to provide symbolic pictures of states of mind.

Whether you live in heaven or hell depends largely upon the kind of thinking you indulge in throughout your day. And, fortunately, you can—using a simple technique—program yourself to rehearse heaven-focused thinking to the benefit of your general state. Think of the doors of hell as swinging doors. You may enter if you wish—and, by the same token, you can also come out as you choose. The way out is to begin thinking thoughts of health, happiness, and success at this very moment.

Allowing the Holism of Our Pain to Heal Us

The word "holistic" is typically associated with health and healing. It generally refers to the natural wholeness that is the result of the balancing and unifying of the body, mind, and spirit. But disease is also a reflection of holism. In fact, disease is the most natural form of holism. Healing is the by-product of following a protocol that reverses the natural, a priori process of disease. By observing the natural course of disease we can construct a map that returns us to a place of homeostasis. Disease is the perfect reflection of nature's if-then decree. If we don't eat enough, then we get malnourished. If we don't sleep enough, then we get tired. If we don't exercise enough, then we get weak. The deductive nature of disease manifests at our deeper mental and emotional levels. If as children we're ignored by our parents, then we'll be more likely to have to contend with fear, shame, and apathy as adults. Moreover, the physics of holism implies an inclusion of "the whole." Therefore, the emotional fear, shame, and apathy that result from years of parental abandonment can also generate physical inflammation in the endocrine system, which is likely to imbalance glucose levels and lead to sugar/carbohydrate addiction, fueling addictive eating patterns and contributing to the risk of obesity. There is no question that by healing the body, heart, mind, and spirit, we heal the whole self—but we also must realize that by diseasing any of these parts, we can also disease the whole self. Once again, it's about our willingness to dig deeper and stretch wider in order to grasp the holism of disease. So long as we insist on attempting to manage our disease at a strictly mechanistic level, the prospect of lasting healing will continue to elude us. Disease may be rooted in the emotional frequencies of our heart, but it ultimately metastasizes to our whole being.

We are born into families, environments, and circumstances that are often chaotic, dysfunctional, abandoning, and abusive. The resulting entropy accompanies us throughout our stages of life, making us emotionally wounded adult children fraught with obsessive-compulsive and addictive tendencies. The all-encompassing holism of this abuse and suffering often stirs compulsive thinking and obsessive control behaviors.

Ever vigilant, our insecure child's mind is constantly scanning its surroundings for any sign of potential threat, real or imagined. If we sense that we're unsafe, we'll adapt our behavior to assert control over our surroundings by seeking pleasure, denying pain, and altering our perceptions.

A friend of mine who's been a pediatric nurse at a major Boston hospital for many years recently shared a disturbing story with me. She explained that the anorexic and bulimic teenage patients in her unit were weighed every morning in an effort to ensure that they were gaining weight. She told me that if they didn't gain weight, they'd be forcibly restrained and force-fed Boost and Ensure through feeding tubes. She then went on to explain that these kids are so afraid of giving up control that they'd go as far as to lubricate two rolls of quarters and place them in their anal cavities, just to add a half pound of body weight. After having heard this story, all I could do was shake my head in disbelief. This sad picture exposes the deepest holistic roots of the dis-ease and pain that ultimately evolved into fear, shame, apathy, and addiction.

In spite of the far-reaching nature of our pain, we must keep in mind that the physics of holism implies a logical duality and balance. If there's a way in, then there's a way out. In fact, the way in could even be seen as a part of the way out. As many of us evolve through our healing process we may eventually come to realize that the very pain that so dis-integrated us was intended to make us whole all along.

This transcendental wisdom is best captured by Kahlil Gibran in his poem "On Pain," in his timeless classic *The Prophet*:

> Much of your pain is self-chosen.
> It is the bitter potion by which the physician within you heals your sick self.[7]

The WHD Emotional Energy Release Exercise

We are an extremely emotionally repressed culture. Because of this repression, our emotional frequencies are generally so highly charged that we become intimidated by the prospect of having to deal with them. The more we deny them, the greater their accumulative force. It is this highly charged repression that forces us to ultimately seek release through alternative behavioral excesses, such as eating and drinking. The key is to demystify these emotions and ultimately to defuse their energetic charge.

This procedure is designed to help release the toxic energies built up from years of repressed fear, shame, and/or apathy. Regardless of which emotional energy we are focused on, it can be effectively released by opening up the heart and grieving it out. It's simply about energy release.

Next, it's important to remember that this is an exercise. It may be an emotional exercise for the internal heart, but it's still an exercise. We exercise our bodies, brains, and minds, but rarely if ever do we exercise our emotional hearts. And when we exercise our bodies, we rely on a support environment, such as an equipped gym, a trainer, a set of headphones, and some kind of music to psych us up. When we exercise our brains and minds, we're also accustomed to a support environment such as a teacher, a classroom, or a laptop. So, in order to effectively exercise our emotional heart, it is equally important to create the proper support environment.

To get set up for the WHD Emotional Energy Release Exercise it is advisable to first establish an appropriate place. It should be a place of privacy and quietude, where you are least likely to be disturbed. Make sure to turn off your cell phone, unplug the landline, and put a Do Not Disturb sign on the door. You should ensure at least twenty to thirty minutes of total privacy. It's also advisable to surround yourself with scrapbooks, mementos, and keepsakes. These are referred to as emotional triggers. These emotional triggers generally make it a bit easier to open up a repressed heart. Finally, be prepared to tune in to some preselected music that plays directly to your heart.

Now that your environment is set, you're ready to begin. Begin listening to the music and slowly filing through your visual triggers. It's essential that you allow your heart to flow freely—laughing, cheering, moaning, groaning, crying, screaming, and yelling as you so feel. Remember, this is intended to be a spontaneous release of feeling expressions passing through your body in the form of highly charged emotional energies.

Once you've engaged in this exercise for thirty minutes, try to allow for an additional ten minutes of quietude to re-center yourself. Also, it's not unusual to be a little bit subdued or feel a little blue for an hour to as much as an entire day or two after. (Do not hesitate to contact a qualified professional counselor for further emotional support.) Once having passed through this brief blue period, you should begin feeling much lighter and clearer. The WHD Emotional Energy Release Exercise should be performed as needed. It is a powerful technique that has proven most effective at defusing the negative driving energies that trigger emotional eating.

THE CHEMISTRY THAT GOVERNS CALORIE-BURNING ENERGY

Metabolism

The alluring promise of the fad diet implies that all one has to do to win at the game of losing weight is simply follow a low-calorie eating plan. But the truth is, dieters are not all equal metabolic performers. Some of us seem to gain weight by just looking at food, while others of us seem to be able to eat continuously, yet never gain weight. It's all about individual metabolism.

Metabolism involves a complex biochemical tapestry of hormones and enzyme catalysts that transform food into fuel. Experts generally agree there are three types of metabolism—slow, balanced, and fast. Slow metabolic types tend to gain weight easily, fast metabolic types struggle to gain weight, and balanced metabolic types usually have efficient metabolisms and fit, healthy bodies.

Our metabolic type is influenced by genetics, age (metabolism slows at the rate of 5 percent per decade after the age of forty), gender (men burn calories more efficiently at rest, for example), ratio of muscle to body mass, thyroid function, type of food consumed, nervous system function, amount of weight carried, and exercise habits. It's all about creating a balance between energy in, energy stored, and energy out. Eighty percent of our population is made up of slow metabolic types.

Generally speaking, slow metabolic types tend to have round, apple-shaped bodies. They are more likely to be sensitive to cold, have low blood pressure, and be less affected by stress. They often lack energy and are deep sleepers, and a majority of them can be classified as having a type B personality. Slow metabolic types are inclined to struggle with weight loss and to gain weight easily. Thus, more than three out of four individuals in our population find it challenging to lose weight, as they are metabolically slow.

Balanced metabolic types have fit, athletic physiques. They generally have a consistent, even flow of energy, have good stamina and healthy eating habits, and are noted for their adaptability during periods of stress. Balanced metabolic types are inclined to have nervous systems that consistently function on an even keel.

Fast metabolic types have lean, pear-shaped bodies, and, while thin, they tend to carry belly fat. Fast types are generally sensitive to heat, have elevated blood pressure, and are overreactive to stress. They have high energy and are fitful sleepers, and a majority of them are classified as having a type A personality. Fast metabolic types tend to lose weight easily and struggle with gaining weight.

We must keep in mind that beyond the material illusion of cells and tissues, we're composed of energy. Each one of us represents a unique manifestation of energy, as does each food we consume. Everything is energy, and all energy is sui generis. Some food energies will activate metabolism for some people but not others. For example, blueberries may activate my metabolism, while slowing yours down—and asparagus may activate my metabolism more than blueberries. As we shall see later, the unique energy interactions between food and people are central to the Whole Health philosophy. In order to maximize our weight loss efficiency we must be willing to evolve beyond the energy-devoid, old-world view of metabolism. By narrowing our view of food as being nothing more than a mass of material proteins, carbohydrates, and fats, we limit our ability to optimize metabolism. We will talk more about the energy aspect of weight loss metabolism later in this book.

What Metabolic Type Are You?

The WHD will take you far beyond the circumscribed material approach to mastering metabolism and weight loss. The unparalleled experience that you are about to encounter will empower you to unleash your highest energy potential for maximum metabolism and weight loss. In the ensuing chapters, you will receive detailed instructions on how to electromagnetically test the energy potential of your thyroid gland. You will also learn a number of bioenergetic protocols that will enable you to optimally balance your metabolic output. In addition, the WHD will teach you how to energy-test your thyroid for positive and negative responses to a variety of foods. This will help you to discover which foods best support your thyroid metabolism and thus your calorie-burning efficiency. Before going on to the energy chapters, it's important that you learn as much about the material aspects of your metabolism as possible. The following questionnaire will help you to decipher your material metabolic type.

The WHD Metabolic Questionnaire

For each question below, circle the response that you feel best describes you.

1. **Your physical shape is:**
   A. Round
   B. Well built
   C. Thin

2. **Your physical constitution is:**
   A. Weak and inactive
   B. Strong and active
   C. Depleted and hyperactive

3. **Your general health is:**
   A. Sickly and allergenic
   B. Good
   C. Run-down

4. **Your resting pulse rate is how many BPMs (beats per minute):**
   A. 50–69
   B. 70–89
   C. 90–110

5. Your blood pressure is:
- A. Low
- B. Normal
- C. High

6. Your blood sugar is:
- A. Low
- B. Normal
- C. High

7. Your body is:
- A. Sensitive to cold and rarely perspires
- B. Rarely too hot or too cold
- C. Sensitive to heat and perspires easily

8. Your mind is:
- A. Underactive
- B. Active
- C. Overactive

9. Your emotional makeup is:
- A. Melancholy and/or depressed
- B. Temperate
- C. Intemperate and/or anxious

10. **Your temperament is:**
    A. Easygoing and pleasant
    B. Self-confident and calm
    C. Impatient and easily agitated

11. **Your personal drive is:**
    A. Low
    B. Average
    C. High

12. **Your energy pace is:**
    A. Slow and deliberate
    B. Even and steady
    C. Fast and labored

13. **Your stress level is:**
    A. Low
    B. Average
    C. High

14. **When you are stressed, you:**
    A. Hit a wall
    B. Recharge
    C. Push through

15. When you first wake up in the morning, you feel:
    A. Exhausted
    B. Refreshed
    C. Unrested and hyper

16. Your energy peaks:
    A. When you first wake up
    B. At midday
    C. In late afternoon or evening

17. Your energy is:
    A. Often highest in the evening
    B. Steady throughout the day
    C. Continually spiking and crashing

18. Your appetite at breakfast is:
    A. Weak
    B. Average
    C. Strong

19. Your appetite at lunch is:
    A. Weak
    B. Average
    C. Strong

20. Your appetite at dinner is:
  A. Weak
  B. Average
  C. Strong

21. You snack in between meals:
  A. Occasionally
  B. Almost never
  C. Frequently

22. Your portion sizes are:
  A. Small
  B. Medium
  C. Large

23. You crave:
  A. Sugars and high-starch carbs
  B. Rarely any cravings
  C. Heavy, fatty, salty foods

24. You gain weight:
  A. Even when you reduce your calorie intake
  B. Rarely—weight rarely fluctuates
  C. Never—weight never fluctuates

25. You lose weight:
    A. With great difficulty
    B. Very rarely
    C. Even though you eat continuously

Once you've completed the questionnaire, you can add up your response totals. If you've circled more A answers, you are a slow oxidizer. If you've circled a higher number of B answers, you are a balanced oxidizer. And if you've circled more C answers, you are a fast oxidizer.

Slow oxidizers should limit their daily intake to:
    1,800 calories
    50 grams of fat (80 percent monounsaturated)
    200 grams of carbohydrates (1 serving of high starch only)

Balanced oxidizers should up their intakes to approximately:
    2,100 calories
    70 grams of fat
    220 grams of carbohydrates

Fast oxidizers, I have a message for you that comes directly from the spirit of my Italian grandmother: **mangia!!!**

More to the point, increase your intake of higher-density fats and high-starch carbohydrates. I suggest 3 tablespoons of coconut and/or olive oil per day added to three servings of some combination of high-starch carbohydrates like brown rice, brown rice pasta, oatmeal, yeast-free/gluten-free toast, potatoes, and sweet potatoes.

Our Metabolic Machinery

A calorie represents a unit of food energy. First defined in 1824 by French physicist and chemist Nicolas Clément, "calorie" is derived from the Latin word *calor*, meaning "heat." The liver is the metabolic powerhouse of the human body—the energy furnace that generates heat from the dietary intake of calories. It is the liver that governs our metabolic rate via the energy-generating process known as anaerobic glycolysis.

The word "glycolysis" refers to the breakdown of glucose (fuel). This action is engaged by a series of enzyme-driven chemical reactions whereby the liver transforms carbohydrates into glucose, the body's primary source of energy. During glycolysis, whatever glucose the body doesn't use is converted into fat. These units of stored fat represent the body's primary source of fuel reserves. When it comes to the biochemical mechanics of calorie burning, the liver works hand in hand with the thyroid gland.

The thyroid is a small, butterfly-shaped gland located at the base of the neck just below the Adam's apple. It produces hormones that regulate the body's metabolic rate, energy, growth, and development. Dr. Stephen Langer, former executive director of the world-renowned Broda Barnes Foundation and author of *Solved: The Riddle of Illness*, tells us that 40 percent of all thyroid disease is presently undiagnosed, resulting in sixty-four common ailments, including athero-sclerosis, depression, arthritis, and type 2 diabetes. For our purposes, we will discuss two major classifications of thyroid disease: hypothyroid (underactive) and hyperthyroid (overactive).

When the thyroid gland is underactive, its metabolic hormone production will also be out of balance, causing a wide range of symptoms. Adenosine tri-phosphate (ATP) is an organic compound present in all living cells that provides energy for the body's vital metabolic processes. If the thyroid gland is underac-tive, and there is an imbalance in the production of thyroid hormone, cells are not able to make ATP for their long-term energy supply.

Hypothyroid is often the primary causal route of chronic fatigue, overweight, and obese conditions. The most common symptoms associated with hypothy-roidism include exhaustion, joint aches, high cholesterol, chronic constipation, dry skin, sensitivity to cold, impaired metabolism, being overweight, and obe-sity. Conversely, symptoms most commonly associated with hyperthyroid in-clude anxiety, nervous energy, rapid heart rate, sensitivity to heat, high blood pressure, being underweight, and the inability to gain weight. When it comes to the issue of calorie-burning efficiency, it's essential for the full complement of thyroid hormones to be in relative balance. The thyroid hormones necessary for a healthy metabolic balance are called T_1, T_2, T_3, T_4, and TSH. The two most important of these hormones are T_3 and T_4. T_4 accounts for 80 percent of the thyroid hormone in the body, but most of the thyroid hormone that enters into the cells is T_3. There are two forms of T_3 and T_4: bound and free. Only about 1 percent of T_3 and 5 percent of T_4 are free. T_4's metabolic effect is slow and long lasting. T_3's effect is fast and short term. Most of the body's T_3 is made in the liver, while T_4 is made in the thyroid gland. These two hormones are key agents in the regulation of cellular metabolism. In order for these hormones to operate at optimal levels, the thyroid requires an adequate supply of certain nutrients: B complex, iron, zinc, selenium, and iodine. When it comes to the assimilation of these vital nutrients, diet is of paramount importance.

Those who've been diagnosed with hypothyroid and are overweight must be very careful to avoid a classification of foods known as progoitrins. Progoitrins are part of the glucosinolate food family, known to suppress the thyroid's all-important iodine uptake. These metabolic saboteurs include cabbage, cauliflower, broccoli, turnips, Brussels sprouts, rutabagas, kale, kohlrabi, mustard greens, spinach, peanuts, soy, walnuts, horseradish, strawberries, mustard greens, and rapeseed oil (canola oil). It's important to underscore that the heat from cooking significantly deactivates the progoitrins from these foods. Therefore, it's imperative that dieters avoid adding any raw progoitrin foods such as broccoli, spinach, or cabbage to their salads. Instead, they should opt for steaming the foods for approximately ten minutes, as the heat destroys goitrogenic compounds. In addition to the issue of progoitrins, those dieters diagnosed with autoimmune disease and/or diseases of the thyroid should bear in mind that mounting evidence indicates that high-gluten grain products such as wheat, barley, and rye should be avoided, as they also place a great deal of stress on thyroid metabolism. Brown rice, amaranth, and quinoa are safer whole-grain options.

The Magnificent Seven Metabolic Hormones

Metabolic hormones are catalysts that regulate virtually every system in the human body. There are anabolic hormones for building and catabolic hormones for breaking things down. Anabolic hormones are responsible for building the body by regulating the ratio of muscle to fat, weight, and general body shape. These hormones are produced by the endocrine system and are intricately orchestrated to play a vital role in determining your body's day-to-day calorie-burning rate. Anabolic hormones are often referred to as "good hormones" because they regulate the burning of fat and the building of muscle. Catabolic hormones are often referred to as "bad hormones" because they destroy muscle, which encourages the body to store fat. In order to be fit and strong, we need to maintain a higher ratio of good hormones to bad hormones. This may sound complicated, but it's actually quite simple. Metabolic hormone balance is largely influenced by the type of foods we eat. A healthy, balanced diet will keep your magnificent seven metabolic hormones in balance:

1. LEPTIN IS OFTEN DESCRIBED BY EXPERTS AS THE SINGLE MOST IMPORTANT HORMONE IN THE HUMAN BODY. Noted author and researcher Byron Richards devoted an entire book to this "superhormone." In *Mastering Leptin*, Richards summarizes the importance of leptin by saying, "Although leptin was not discovered until 1994, what first seemed like a key hormone that regulated the response to starvation soon became the superstar of hormones. Leptin is in control; all other hormones answer up to leptin."[1] Leptin is the energy broker for the body, literally providing the energy currency to make

metabolism work. It is secreted by fat cells contained within the body's white adipose tissue—the unsightly fat that accumulates in all the wrong places like the abdomen, buttocks, and thighs. Leptin is a messenger molecule that communicates with every cell between the brain and body. Whenever there is a breakdown in this communication process, caused by aging, stress, and/or poor diet, it results in uncontrollable food cravings, addictive and compulsive behavior, and weight gain. When the body becomes biochemically imbalanced, the brain loses its ability to effectively register leptin levels. This ultimately leads to a resistance to the hormone. Once the body has built up a resistance to leptin, it will then tend to overcompensate by producing and absorbing too much of the hormone. This entire leptin resistance quagmire begins with prolonged stress and poor diet. Prolonged stress leads to adrenaline resistance, which causes fat accumulation around the midsection. Poor diet leads to insulin resistance, resulting in general fat storage, chronic fatigue, insomnia, and acute inflammation. As you can plainly see, once leptin resistance sets in, metabolism will spiral out of control. The good news is, no matter how far this cycle of leptin resistance has progressed, it takes only twenty-one days to rebalance. Twenty-one days of fewer total calories, a 4:3 protein-to-high-starch-carbohydrate ratio, no snacks, and an effective commitment to stress management will enable you to regain your all-important leptin balance. By keeping your leptin in balance you'll be keeping your other magnificent six in balance.

2. GHRELIN IS A HORMONAL SIGNALING MOLECULE THAT'S PRODUCED BY SPECIALIZED CELLS IN THE SMALL INTESTINE, STOMACH, PANCREAS, AND

THYROID. It tells the brain when the body is hungry, and it has been shown to increase the accumulation of harmful lipids in the tissues of the abdominal wall. You might think of ghrelin as the "belly fat" hormone. There is a close relationship between ghrelin and leptin. When leptin is out of balance, ghrelin also goes out of balance, throwing the brain and the body into a vicious tailspin. Now, instead of merely signaling the brain that the body is hungry when it is really hungry, ghrelin transmits continuous hunger signals by stimulating the hypothalamus to increase levels of a thirty-six-amino-acid endocannabinoid protein called neuropeptide Y. Researchers have recently discovered that high protein intake lowers ghrelin levels and high carbohydrate intake elevates them. By increasing the hormone glucagon, an insulin antagonist protein drives up our calorie-burning energy. On the other hand, high-starch carbs drive up insulin, which tends to increase fat storage.

3. NEUROPEPTIDE Y SENDS HUNGER SIGNALS THROUGHOUT THE BRAIN AND BODY, AND IF IT IS IMBALANCED BY CONFUSING SIGNALS FROM LEPTIN AND GHRELIN, IT WILL DRIVE UP THE BODY'S CRAVINGS FOR FATTY, SALTY, AND SUGARY FOODS. As long as leptin levels are low, ghrelin levels will increase and neuropeptide Y levels will remain high, making it virtually impossible for your brain to turn off the appetite switch. Once again, it all starts with leptin. Follow the leptin dietary suggestions to keep your magnificent seven in balance.

4. INSULIN IS A HORMONE THAT'S RELEASED BY THE PANCREAS TO HELP REGULATE BLOOD SUGAR LEVELS. Whenever we eat an excess of sugar or

high-starch carbohydrates such as bread, pasta, rice, or potatoes, the body converts the sugar and starch into glucose, which it immediately releases into the bloodstream. Next, insulin release keeps blood glucose from rising too high, by either burning it as fuel or storing it as fat. When more is consumed than can be used, fat stores rise. It's not too hard to see how vital the proper maintenance of insulin is to weight loss and fitness. It all comes down to insulin—it's either fueling us for action or downloading us with fat storage.

5. GLUCAGON IS THE INSULIN ANTAGONIST. In order for metabolism to operate at its highest level, insulin and glucagon should be in balance. Where insulin is designed to lower blood sugar levels, glucagon elevates low blood sugar. Glucagon offsets the body's low blood sugar fuel outages by tapping into the liver's stored reserves of fat for backup energy. Thus, where insulin stores fat, glucagon incinerates it as fuel. So, in simple terms, the more sugar and high starch we consume, the more insulin we secrete, and the more fat we store. On the other hand, the more protein we eat, the more glucagon we produce, and the more calories we burn. Of course, as we've already stated, balance is important. A 4:3 protein-to-carbohydrate ratio will help you to maintain a balanced magnificent seven.

6. CORTISOL IS A PRIMARY STEROID HORMONE PRODUCED BY THE ADRENAL GLANDS DURING PERIODS OF BOTH ACUTE AND CHRONIC STRESS. Without cortisol, our bodies would simply not be able to adapt to the demands

of stress. Cortisol supports our self-protective, fight-or-flight mobilization response. It readies us to make the necessary short-term moves with swifter, greater efficiency. Keep in mind: I said short term! The stress state produces a lot of energy, but it also requires a lot of energy. There's a great deal of biochemical wear and tear here. I once saw a study concluding that the average human body is physiologically designed to adapt to stress for no more than 15 percent of its lifetime. I'm guessing that most of us are running just a wee bit over that mark. So what's the worst that could happen if we were to find ourselves in a state of stress for more than 15 percent of our lifetime? More to the point, what's the worst that could happen to our metabolism?

Due to the fact that our bodies are designed to contend with only short-term stress and cortisol production, long-term stress causes problems with blood sugar, blood pressure, and fat storage, giving rise to a condition known as "metabolic syndrome." Metabolic syndrome results in a high waist-to-hip ratio, with an excessive accumulation of abdominal body fat. Besides increasing risks for heart disease, diabetes, stroke, arthritis, fibromyalgia, lupus, asthma, and allergies, metabolic syndrome increases cravings for salt, sugar, and high-starch carbohydrates—all of which contribute to overweight and obesity. I've discovered that there's a very complicated relationship between the adrenal glands and the thyroid gland when it comes to stress. The more stress we experience, the more mobilizing, fight-or-flight hormones like cortisol and adrenaline we produce. The greater the concentrations of fight-or-flight hormones we produce, the more we overwork our thyroid gland. The more we overwork our thyroid gland, the less efficient it is at regulating our metabolism. Anyone who doesn't overeat, yet has an excess accumulation of abdominal body fat, needs to focus on reducing their stress levels. They might consider meditation, yoga, tai chi, or qigong. Cortisol teaches us that diet alone is not the answer. The stress–cortisol connection reminds us that the body, mind, and spirit are always working together.

7. TESTOSTERONE IS A HORMONE THAT MOST PEOPLE KNOW AT LEAST A LITTLE SOMETHING ABOUT. But it does much more than merely tune up our sex machine. Testosterone is also our preeminent muscle builder. In order to be firm and strong, with a low fat-to-muscle ratio, our bodies have to be sufficiently supplied with this all-important hormone. According to recent studies, obese men given testosterone shots have lost significant amounts of weight in short periods of time. Testosterone is a superior metabolic activator that has even been shown to strengthen heart function. The most important dietary advice for maintaining healthy testosterone levels is to make sure that our diet is composed of at least 30 percent fat, from healthy, monounsaturated, and medium-chain saturated lipids. Extra-virgin olive oil, avocado, and coconut milk are among the best options. Also, be sure to get a minimum of seven and a half hours of sleep each night. Inadequate sleep markedly decreases our body's production of anabolic hormones like testosterone. Sleep represents our most efficient way to recover from stress. Excessive stress kills metabolism!

Our "Super" Metabolic Regulators

In 1930, pharmacologist Charles Leib and gynecologist Raphael Kurzrok first identified vital components of human semen called prostaglandins. Prostaglandins are a group of super, hormonelike cell mediators, derived from fatty acids that perform important functions that have extremely powerful effects on the human body.

When Swedish physiologist Ulf von Euler and researcher M. W. Goldblatt first isolated human prostaglandins from seminal fluid in 1935, the stage was set for the world's first introduction to a much broader understanding of inflammation as a disease-producing chemistry. Von Euler's lifelong research in this area earned him the Nobel Prize in Medicine in 1970. Around that same time, researchers Sune K. Bergström and Bengt Samuelsson further detailed exactly how fatty acids set up inflammatory pathways in the body. The merger of their prostaglandin research with that of John R. Vane resulted in a Nobel Prize in Medicine in 1982.

Today, prostaglandins are referred to as eicosanoids, which are believed to act as superhormones in virtually all body systems. Many experts now think of eicosanoids as the most powerful biochemical agents in the human body. In fact, they are signaling molecules that initiate many of our most vital cellular chains of command and communication. Eicosanoids might be thought of as the field generals of our cells, as they order them on their inflammatory and anti-inflammatory missions throughout the global body network. The importance of this process cannot be overstated and, in fact, eicosanoid programming is a matter of life and death.

Some experts now believe that nearly 75 percent of the 14,199 coded diseases presently known are caused by inflammatory eicosanoid programming. This chronic inflammatory disease process currently affects 130 million Americans. While it may seem hard to believe, this all-important, life-and-death chemistry actually begins with diet.

Foods produce essential fatty acids. All fatty acids produce one of three categories of eicosanoids: neutral, inflammatory, or anti-inflammatory. Fatty acids are the raw materials from which inflammatory eicosanoids are produced. Therefore, you could say that a vast majority of disease is caused by the overconsumption of bad fats. Thus, many biochemically triggered diseases can be successfully modulated by therapeutic diet. Diet-induced inflammation has been causally implicated in cancer, heart disease, type 2 diabetes, rheumatoid arthritis, and lupus, among others. In addition, conditions that lead to overweight and obesity are also representative of eicosanoid imbalances. Inflammation assaults the immune system and confuses the metabolism. It is virtually impossible to lose weight and be fit if your body is inflamed.

Hidden food allergens, red meat, dairy products, egg yolks, peanuts, processed sugar products, and high-starch carbohydrates—as well as foods containing omega-6 oils—are among those foods that produce high levels of arachidonic fatty acid, the fatty acid from which all disease-producing inflammatory eicosanoids are manufactured in the body. Anti-inflammatory eicosanoids, on the other hand, are manufactured from the healthy alpha-linolenic acid, commonly found in wild fatty fish, soy products, shelled walnuts, flaxseeds, pumpkin seeds, and organic produce. Eat plenty of these foods for super metabolic regulation.

The Six Keys to Resetting Metabolism

Only when our metabolic superhormones are in balance will our calorie-burning potential operate at peak efficiency levels. Here are six important recommendations that will help to reset and balance your metabolic superhormones.

1. INCREASE PROTEIN. For starters, we must maintain a 40:30:30 ratio of protein to carbohydrate to fat in our diet. This ratio enables us to produce higher levels of glucagon and lower levels of insulin, thus supporting our body's efforts to burn fat more efficiently. Overweight, obese people tend to consume a higher starch to-protein dietary ratio.

2. AVOID BEDTIME SNACKING. It is important to leave a twelve-hour gap between our final bite of dinner and our first bite of the next morning's breakfast. This twelve-hour gap supports our body's efforts to produce a sufficient supply of leptin for the next day. Remember, when leptin levels go down, insulin levels rise, thus driving up fat storage.

3. AVOID DAYTIME SNACKING. Generally try to avoid appreciable snacking between meals. It takes a significant amount of digestive energy to break food down. If, shortly after completing a meal, we indulge in additional calorie intake, our bodies will be robbed of the required energy to resupply themselves with leptin and glucagon.

4. RELEASE YOUR STRESS ENERGY. Engage in three minutes of deep breathing twice daily. This will serve to curb your body's production of stress hormones, namely adrenaline, enabling you to reverse adrenaline resistance, the principal saboteur of metabolic superhormones. I've been reminding my patients for years that the body and mind have only so much energy to spend. Whatever energy we commit to stress will ultimately take away from what's required to repair and engage our calorie-burning machinery.

5. GET YOUR SLEEP. Try to get sound, uninterrupted sleep every night. Studies have shown that our bodies require seven hours and twenty minutes of sound sleep every night to recover from the stresses of the day. When you consider that adrenaline resistance is the archenemy of a healthy metabolism, sound sleep recovery from the ravages of daily stress is essential for optimal calorie burning. You won't lose weight if you don't sleep. If you suffer from chronic insomnia you might try supplementing with 250 mg of magnesium taurate and 40 drops of passionflower tincture in 3 ounces of water before bedtime.

6. REGULATE YOUR PH. One of our most important metabolic health cycles is that of pH (potential hydrogen). Generally speaking, acidity results from high stress and poor diet and is a basic indicator of poor cellular oxygenation and ill health. Acid pH is most readily determined by urinating on color-coated, .067 calibrated Nitrazine strips. The total pH range is measured in tenths from 5.0–8.0. Healthy pH balance is between 6.4 and 6.8. A score below 6.4 is too acidic, indicating oxygen deficiency. A score over 6.8 is too alkaline,

indicating enzyme deficiency. Speaking strictly in terms of calorie-burning potential, all you need to know about pH is that it determines the body's rate of cellular oxygenation. As I'm sure you know, without sufficient oxygen, you can't have fire. And so it is with calorie burning—oxygen feeds our calorie-burning fire as well. A blood pH of 7.45 produces 64.9 percent more oxygen than a blood pH of 7.30. If you want to burn calories you have to maintain a urinary pH between 6.4 and 6.8. Acidosis ravages metabolism! The best way to ensure that your lifestyle supports alkalinity is to consume eight servings of vegetables and fruits and a minimum of 40 ounces of pure water per day. Chronically acidic pH may require supplementation with ¼ teaspoon of baking soda in 4 ounces of water before bed until corrected.

Turning on Your Metabolic Gene Machinery

There are those who would blame the current chronic weight gain and obesity problems on genetic determinism. Researchers tell us that events and exposures occurring during critical developmental periods of life can act as triggers for metabolic diseases such as obesity.

Epidemiological studies of adults exposed in utero to calorie restriction during the Dutch Hunger Winter during World War II show that they were statistically more likely to become overweight and obese. Epigenetic experts believe that things like in utero calorie restriction, tobacco exposure, nutrient intake, circulating hormones, and environmental pollutants are among the many events and exposures that ultimately play a significant role in gene-expression programming that can lead to obesity.

Researchers have discovered that when human fetuses were exposed to endocrine-disrupting chemicals such as dioxin, dioxin-like compounds, DDT, and pharmaceuticals, there were changes in the babies' genes that altered their metabolic function, predisposing them to obesity.

So, long before we're born, our gene mapping system is actively responding to its environment. This ultimately has a powerful influence over our metabolic demand for calories as adults. But this developmental plasticity serves as a reminder that genetically we're really not all that hardwired. We've been taught that our genes are immutable, and while it's true that our genes can't be altered, their behavior can be. Thus, in utero plasticity influences that can work against us can also be reformatted so as to work in our favor as adults. While it's obvious that things like in utero calorie restriction, tobacco exposure, and exposure to endocrine-disrupting chemicals can program our genes to crave fat, sugar, and a high calorie intake, it's also been proven that positive influences such as calorie restriction and high antioxidant nutrient intake can help reverse negative gene expression. Science continues to discover a myriad of positive gene expression influences.

In 1995, a team of researchers made a presentation at the Proceedings of the National Academy of Sciences sharing the remarkable results of their animal studies showing that fasting had an antiobesity gene expression effect on obese animals.[2] Then in 2005, Japanese researchers discovered that antioxidant-rich cocoa has the potential to reverse gene obesity expression in animals.[3] In 2007, Chinese scientists discovered the antiobesity effect of an antioxidant nutrient found in green tea called epigallocatechin gallate (EGCG) on lipid metabolism and adipokine gene expression.[4] Additionally, in 2013 Spanish researchers found that apple polyphenol antioxidants were able to reverse adipocyte gene expression in rats.[5]

The human body produces a gene for every occasion. We produce taste genes, texture genes, appetite genes, glucose genes, insulin genes—fat genes and thin genes. Unbeknownst to us, we're continually turning different genes on and off like light switches. Our diets, behaviors, and even our thoughts profoundly influence the on/off buttons of the genes that control much of our weight loss potential.

Researchers at the University of Texas Southwestern Medical Center recently discovered an important protein that turns genes on and off and plays a vital role in the regulation of metabolism. The protein, called X-box binding protein 1, or Xbp1, is believed to regulate both insulin sensitivity and leptin signaling, making it extremely important for appetite control and blood sugar management.[6]

The scientists discovered that the enhanced expression of the Xbp1 gene in animals fed a high-fat diet served as protection against the onset of obesity and diabetes. On average, the mice that had the Xbp1 gene turned on were 30 percent thinner than the mice without the gene support, which were fed the same high-fat diet. The researchers noted that the manipulation of this gene increased metabolic function in the hypothalamus gland. It also influenced areas of the brain that control liver glucose production. They reported that the gene sent satiety signals to the hypothalamus, curbing appetite, and to the liver, improving blood sugar efficiency. The recurring story here is that calorie-burning genes can be turned on and calorie-storing genes can be turned off. Ironically, foods are what turn the switches.

High-protein, high-fiber, good-fat, chemical-free foods, and antioxidant-rich spices have been shown—in study after study—to turn on calorie-burning genes, while turning off calorie-storing gene expression. Avocado, salmon, flax-seeds, grapefruit, egg whites, olive oil, chili peppers, and ginger have all demon-strated the potential to turn off "fat genes" and turn on "thin genes."

Of course, the way we use these foods is also of the utmost importance. Gene expression research has shown that frequent snacking, especially before bed, turns off our thin gene switch. Missing meals—or "gapping"—has also been shown to turn off thin genes, as it is believed to lower leptin levels.

Genes have long been known as powerful agents of change, but we're now just beginning to understand that there's a less fixed, more "plastic" side to their behavior that allows us a greater degree of programming access. What we eat, when we eat it, how we think, and how often we think it all influence our met-abolic gene expression.

Reprogramming Your Brain for Metabolic Efficiency

Neuroscience has recently discovered that a part of the brain called the lateral hypothalamus is a key regulator of our appetite and feeding patterns. This is largely due to its production of neuronal hormones—like hypocretins, orexins, and dopaminergics—associated with arousal, reward, and stability. This neuro-nal hormone network projects widely throughout the entire brain, but is most specifically involved with the regulation of the amygdala (stress) and the nucleus accumbens (reward) responses. The hypothalamus controls hunger, thirst, satiety, and stress regulation and is therefore highly relevant to our understanding of the brain's addiction mechanisms.

This brain network and the neurotransmission pathways it presides over are directly responsible for the recall of negative emotional memories associated with addiction withdrawal and the prompting of positive emotional memories associated with addiction cues. You might say that those among us who are more "lateral hypothalamic/amygdala/nucleus accumbens–brain dominant" are predominantly operating out of our addictive brain centers. The $64,000 question then would be, is it possible to reprogram our brain dominance to beat food addiction and increase our prospects for weight loss? More specifically, the question might be: is it possible to shift from midbrain dominance to pineal gland dominance? And if so, how?

The pineal gland, or epiphysis cerebri, is a pea-sized endocrine gland located directly between the two brain hemispheres. This tiny gland, shaped like a pinecone, works in concert with the hypothalamus to regulate our hunger, thirst, stress, and aging. It has often been referred to as the "third eye," as it's believed to represent transformational human visionary potential. René Descartes referred to the pineal gland as "the seat of the soul."

When the pineal gland is healthy and functioning optimally, it produces melatonin, serotonin, and pinoline hormones to help the brain more efficiently regulate stress, recovery, and addiction. Moreover, many experts are now asserting that the pineal gland holds the key to our potential transcendence of addiction.

Researchers have recently demonstrated a direct connection between a powerful neurochemical agent and a transformative modulator of human consciousness known as dimethyltryptamine (DMT) within the pineal gland. DMT, a substance naturally produced in plants, animals, and humans, is presently being studied for its consciousness-expanding, antiaddiction potential. A growing number of experts now believe that human DMT deficiency, caused by fat-laden diets, fluoride consumption, and stress, have made our brains increasingly susceptible to addiction by shutting down our antiaddictive pineal response. Therefore, it is believed that we can support our brain's antiaddiction chemistry by enhancing DMT absorption efficiency. The WHD suggests the following recommendations to increase DMT absorption efficiency and reprogram your brain for weight loss:

1. Lower total fat consumption to 30 percent of total calories, 80 percent of which should be monounsaturated.
2. Eat only USDA organic products, free-range (responsibly farmed) meats, and wild fish.
3. Avoid fluoridated drinking water, toothpaste, and mouthwash. Fluoride consumption increases the toxic calcification of the pineal gland.
4. Supplement with 1 serrapeptase 120,000 unit capsule three times daily on an empty stomach.
5. Supplement with 1 menaquinone (MK-7) 100 mcg capsule twice daily on an empty stomach.
6. Practice prayer, meditation, yoga, and/or tai chi regularly.

Trace Minerals for Metabolic Support

There are a number of viable nutritional strategies for optimizing metabolic output, but there are none better than efficient mineral management. "Minerals comprise approximately four percent of our total body weight and include macro and micro elements," writes Dr. David L. Watts. "The macro-elements are those found in the body in high concentrations, such as calcium, phosphorus, sodium, potassium, and sulfur. Micro-elements, or trace elements, are present in low concentrations and include elements such as chromium, vanadium, selenium, lithium, and manganese. Their functions range from providing structural support in the formation of bones and teeth, to maintaining the acid base balance, nerve conduction, muscle contraction, and enzyme functions. Some minerals participate in hundreds of biochemical processes, while others participate in only limited functions. Their role in health and disease has just recently been recognized, such as their involvement in the prevention of cancer, immune regulation, chronic degenerative disease, eating, and even emotions. In the words of the late Dr. Henry Schroeder, 'Minerals are the basic spark plugs in the chemistry of life, on which the exchanges of energy in the combustion of food's building of living tissue depend.' This statement emphasizes the extreme importance of essential minerals in biological systems for optimal function and health."[7] This is especially true for optimal metabolic function.

Virtually every food we consume and every thought we think influences our mineral profile, which in turn influences our metabolism. Slow metabolic mineral patterns reveal stored tissue elevations of calcium, magnesium, and copper. Moreover, those who struggle with weight loss are inclined to have a very high calcium-to-potassium ratio. This is especially troubling when you consider that so many of us have been coerced by the medical orthodoxy to freely consume dairy products and to supplement our diets with calcium. On the other hand, fast metabolic mineral patterns reflect very low levels of calcium and magnesium and very elevated levels of sodium and potassium. Fast metabolic types tend to exhibit particularly low calcium-to-potassium ratios.

Our stored mineral ratio profiles are a reflection of both cause and effect. They reveal our constitutional tendencies regarding functions such as calorie burning, but they're also important keys to changing our calorie-burning potential. In short, if you are overweight and have struggled with weight loss, it's very likely that your stored tissue calcium and magnesium levels are abnormally high. It's also likely your calcium-to-potassium ratio is abnormally elevated. If you were to obtain a mineral test to confirm these results, you could then supplement with minerals to correct these imbalances and improve your metabolic function. The WHD highly recommends that the dieter consider obtaining a trace mineral analysis (TMA). This important and affordable test provides people with a detailed account of their minerals and mineral ratios, which can assist you in the management of your minerals for maximum metabolic output.

TMA is a very simple procedure that analyzes human tissue. The Environmental Protection Agency (EPA) and most medical communities worldwide consider human hair to be an acceptable tissue for biological monitoring. It is the perfect medium, as it readily absorbs all trace element minerals. Hair contains seven layers of protein, and the third-innermost layer, or cortex, is mostly made up of carotene and approximately 58 percent carbon. This cortex layer, therefore, serves as a perfect repository for stored minerals. TMA laboratories analyze hair cortex mineral status by means of atomic absorption spectroscopy and plasma emission spectroscopy. This refraction of atomic light through the cortex sample reveals the mineral makeup with great precision. Assuming that your TMA test has confirmed that you have a slow metabolic mineral pattern, you may then want to supplement with nutrients that enable you to balance out your profile and maximize your metabolism for greater weight loss efficiency. Generally speaking, to counteract a slow metabolic mineral pattern, you'd want to increase sodium, potassium, and iron. In addition, you may also want to supplement with vitamin A, vitamin E, and the B complex vitamins, as they are representative of nutrients that will stimulate the body's metabolic processes. Below is a list of the WHD's specific supplement recommendations for those interested in balancing their slow metabolic mineral patterns:

Sodium ascorbate: 1,000 mg per day
Liquid potassium citrate: 1 teaspoon (99 mg) twice weekly
Floravital liquid iron: 1 tablespoon per day
Gamma E: 600 IU per day
B complex: 50 mg twice daily
Vitamin A: 10,000 IU per day

TMA can help you better manage your minerals for optimal metabolic output.

NOTE: While this list represents general, safe recommendations, it is advised that one should consult with a qualified health care professional before beginning any nutritional supplement program.

A Key Metabolic Vitamin

According to a joint National Institutes of Health and University of Cincinnati study, recently presented at a meeting of the International Society of Endocrinology and the Endocrine Society, vitamin D treatment alters the brain and brain chemistry in such a way as to improve weight and blood sugar control in obese animals.[8]

The research team gave the most active potent form of vitamin D, called 1,25-dihydroxyvitamin D3, to a control group of obese male rats, through a surgically inserted feeding tube. Both glucose testing and vitamin D monitoring were consistently administered over a twenty-eight-day test period. The rats were split up into two groups, a control group and a vitamin D group. The rats in the group that received vitamin D consumed nearly three times less food and lost 24 percent of their total body weight. The vitamin D group also experienced improved glucose tolerance, revealing an improved efficiency regarding insulin sensitivity and body response to sugar. The research team underscored the fact that vitamin D deficiency tends to commonly occur in obese patients with type 2 diabetes. They were also quick to point out that their study results were in no way intended to minimize the importance of diet and exercise. In order to control weight and blood sugar, vitamin D supplementation should accompany a healthy diet and exercise program.

Similar results were found by researchers at Creighton University in Omaha, Nebraska. "Researchers tapped into a huge international database, accessing the genetic profiles of more than 42,000 people. Scientists noted whether a person harbored any of 12 genetic variants associated with being overweight. Not surprisingly, people with these variants were more likely to be obese than those without them. People with these obesity-associated gene variants were also apt to have low vitamin D levels."[9]

Their data further suggested that losing weight could potentially reverse vitamin D deficiency in obese people. These experts theorize that the reason vitamin D seems to play such a significant role in weight gain, obesity, and blood sugar is because vitamin D is fat soluble and appears to sequester within the body's fat cells.

In yet another study, published in April 2014 in the *American Journal of Clinical Nutrition*, researchers discovered that vitamin D may be associated with weight loss in postmenopausal women. A research team at the Fred Hutchinson Cancer Research Center evaluated the results of vitamin D supplementation administered to overweight women ages fifty to seventy-five with a low vitamin D baseline. The study matched up twelve months of vitamin D supplementation (2,000 IU per day) compared with placebos on changes in body weight and composition—as well as metabolic markers such as insulin—during a supervised dietary period. Those women with higher vitamin D levels showed greater improvements in body composition compared with women of lower vitamin D levels. Those women with the highest vitamin D levels lost an average of nineteen pounds during the twelve months, and the placebo group lost an average of twelve pounds during that same period.[10]

The WHD advises that those who are interested in losing weight consider having their vitamin D levels checked by their provider and replenished if needed.

A Fat That Stimulates Metabolic Fat Burning

After years of relative obscurity, an adipose tissue known as "brown fat" is suddenly garnishing a great deal of attention in the nutritional world. Research has shown that leaner, fitter bodies tend to have more brown fat. Overweight and obese bodies, on the other hand, typically have a higher concentration of "white fat." White fat represents the undesirable stored energy that most of the world is trying to lose. Some researchers believe that brown fat is actually more like muscle than fat, as it actually burns the bad white fat when metabolically stimulated.

Nature's plan was for brown fat to keep the human body warm. Scientists have discovered that people who live in colder climates produce more brown fat during the winter months. Experts believe that taking cold showers and sleeping with the window open on cold winter nights are among the best ways to increase brown fat production in the body and step up calorie-burning potential.

Unfortunately, of the twenty to forty pounds of total fat in the average human body, only two to three ounces of it is brown fat. However, that minuscule amount of brown fat has the potential to incinerate up to 500 calories a day! That's exactly why researchers are currently in search of new drugs to stimulate our production of brown fat.

Most of the body's brown fat is strategically located near the heart, around the neck and chest, between the shoulder blades, and in the retroperitoneal region behind the kidneys. These zones allow the brown fat direct access to the body's most active circulation centers, enabling it to convert its energy into metabolic heat. It's this thermogenic effect that accounts for the calorie-burning dynamic of brown fat.

Physical movement, playfulness, and stimulating environments, in addition to exposure to cold, have been shown to increase the production of brown fat in animal studies. In fact, after only one month of being in a stimulating environment, animals had significantly less visceral fat when compared to animals in a less stimulating, controlled environment. It seems that when their minds were creatively excited by a diversely enriched environment, their brain production of a protein called BDNF, or brain-derived neurotrophic factor—shown to dramatically accelerate brown fat production and white fat incineration—was also increased.

A number of recent studies have demonstrated that brown fat has a profound influence not only on weight loss but on general health. Researchers at the University of Texas Medical Branch at Galveston discovered that brown fat supports blood sugar function, insulin sensitivity, and optimal metabolism, as well as the incineration of arterial fat stores. These scientists showed that mild exposure to cold for periods of five to eight hours elevated body energy, increased eradication of excess sugar from the bloodstream, and enhanced insulin sensitivity in tissue stores—supporting the theory that brown fat may act as an antidiabetic agent in the human body.[11]

Ten Pharmaceutical Medicines
That Can Sabotage Metabolism

If you're serious about losing weight the WHD way and you're presently on medication, you may want to have a conversation with your doctor. Here's a list of ten common medications that have been shown to interfere with weight loss:

1. ALLEGRA. A study performed in 2010 established that those subjects taking prescription antihistamines such as Allegra were up to 55 percent more likely to be overweight than those not taking the drugs.[12] Some experts believe that histamine can disrupt an important metabolic enzyme in the brain that regulates appetite.

2. DEPAKOTE. According to an epilepsy study performed in 2007, 24 percent of men and 44 percent of women who took Depakote for one year gained eleven or more pounds.[13]

3. PAXIL. Paxil is one of the more effective anxiety medicines, but if you've gained weight while using it, you should talk with your doctor about switching to a more weight-loss-friendly SSRI. Experts appear uncertain as to why, but Paxil does appear to interfere with metabolism and weight loss for some patients.

4. PROZAC. Recent studies have shown that over time Prozac may cause weight gain for some. Many experts theorize that the reason for this is that the drug

may slow metabolism and increase appetite. Some physicians who suspect this problem often switch their patients to Wellbutrin, which has been associated with weight loss.

5. REMERON. Due to its antihistamine effect, this antidepressant is suspected to significantly increase appetite and weight gain.

6. ZYPREXA. According to a 2005 study, 30 percent of the subjects who were put on this atypical antipsychotic drug gained 7 percent of their body weight in eighteen months. Once again, the antihistamine activity is suspected to cause weight gain for some.

7. PREDNISONE. Long-term use of both oral and inhaled forms of steroids have long been known as weight gain triggers. A number of studies attempting to discover weight gain strategies for severely underweight HIV patients and burn victims were among the first to make this connection. Researchers have discovered that steroids work in much the same way as antithyroid medications.

8. THORAZINE. Medical experts have known since as far back as the mid-1950s that this antipsychotic drug has a proclivity to cause weight gain.

9. ELAVIL. This most popular TCA (tricyclic antidepressant) medication on the market today, primarily prescribed for migraine headaches, depression, and anxiety disorders, has become associated with marked weight gain. In fact

it's been estimated that as many as 50 percent of its users discontinue treatment solely due to its weight gain side effects.

10. NEXIUM AND PREVACID. Heartburn medicines such as Nexium and Prevacid have been shown to cause weight gain. Before recommending these medications, a growing number of physicians are now advising their patients to adjust their diets accordingly.

NOTE: If you're presently taking any of these medications, **the WHD urges you not to discontinue!** Instead, you're advised to have a conversation with your doctor so that you can express your weight loss concerns.

Common Household Toxins That Are Bad for Your Metabolism

Chances are good that your home environment is riddled with sources of toxic chemicals capable of seriously impairing your thyroid function. Experts estimate the average American is routinely exposed to more than six thousand toxic chemicals, many of which are endocrine disrupters that can create thyroid havoc. It seems as though there's no stopping the chemicals that are at last stopping us. As an old Monsanto commercial once put it, "Without chemicals, life itself would be impossible."[14]

For starters, nearly all of our homes are saturated with flame-retardant organobromine compounds, called polybromated diphenyl ethers (PBDEs).

PBDEs emit vaporous toxins that are released from sources such as motor vehicle upholstery, electronics, plastics, carpets, textiles, building insulation, and polyurethane foam in furnishings.

Experts say PBDEs are likely present in the bloodstreams of up to 97 percent of U.S. residents, at levels twenty times higher than in people in Europe. Studies have found that a tenfold increase in PBDEs is capable of depressing thyroid-stimulating hormone (TSH) by nearly 17 percent, significantly increasing the risk for hyperthyroid disease. When low TSH levels appear alongside normal T4 levels, it is an indication of hyperthyroidism, an endocrine condition that is especially problematic during pregnancy.

Also, a recent seven-year epidemiological study of nearly four thousand people, performed at the University of Exeter and the Peninsula Medical School, has linked thyroid disease to perfluorooctanoic acid (PFOA) exposure. PFOA is a toxic chemical typically found in nonstick cookware, stain- and water-resistant fabric, and carpet coatings. The analytical data produced by the researchers showed a direct statistical link between high serum concentrations of PFOAs and thyroid disease.[15]

The World Health Organization recently presented some very troubling landmark study results revealing that the average American is commonly exposed to a class of chemicals called endocrine-disrupting chemicals (EDCs) that can lead to thyroid cancer and obesity. EDCs are most commonly found in products containing bisphenol A (BPA), like plastic water bottles, plastic milk containers, plastic microwave ovenware, and the lining of canned foods. Similar endocrine results were recently found by a University of Michigan epidemiological study of 1,346 adults and 329 adolescents. Generally, higher concentrations of BPAs were associated with a higher likelihood of thyroid disruption.[16]

The WHD Metabolic Detox Protocol

The WHD holds that if we want our thyroid to burn calories efficiently, then we need to cleanse it of its metabolic toxins at least once a year. We must remember that toxic exposures are accumulative, so it is most important that we occasionally cleanse our calorie-burning machinery.

There are many and varied forms of nutritional detoxification. There are a variety of intestine, liver, lymph, and blood detoxification programs that are all designed to cleanse the body in order to bring it back to some semblance of homeostasis. The WHD Five-Day Metabolic Detox Diet and Supplement Plan is a five-day cleansing program designed to rid the body of some of the chemical toxins that disrupt metabolism.

Detoxification is the metabolic process of removing unwanted compounds from the body, such as environmental contaminants, inflammatory hormones, endotoxins, and single-cell bacteria. The blood and lymph systems are extremely important detox transport pathways, but the predominant detox organs are the liver, intestines, and kidneys. These all-important pathways and organs follow a sequence called Phase 1, 2, and 3. These three phases are representative of powerful enzyme systems that keep the vital organ pathways active and clear during detoxification.

Phase 1 enzymes break toxins down into chemicals that can be metabolized by Phase 2 enzymes. It's accurate to say that Phase 1 sets up Phase 2. Phase 2 enzymes are then able to attach the toxins to water-soluble sites in order to prepare them for the next phase of transiting and release. Finally, Phase 3 enzymes deliver the toxins to cells that, in turn, transport them to bile or urine for excretion.

As the body sequences through each separate enzyme phase of detoxification, it is important to supplement with specific nutrients capable of supporting each organ system. For an effective metabolic detox, a specially designed nutritional supplement protocol should accompany a metabolic diet.

The WHD Five-Day Metabolic Detox Diet and Supplement Plan

Repeat the following recommendations for five consecutive days.

Breakfast
MORNING SMOOTHIE

■ Blend together:

½ cup berries of any kind

2 tablespooons ground flaxseeds

1 tablespoon ProFibe

1 tablespoon ProGreens

12 ounces pure water

Supplement with:

Barberry root tincture: 20 drops in 4 ounces water

N-acetyl cysteine: 500 mg capsule

Alpha-lipoic acid: 100 mg capsule

Citrus bioflavonoid complex: 500 mg tablet

Jarro-Dophilus EPS probiotic: 1 capsule

Jarrow Curcumin 95: 500 mg capsule

Midmorning Snack

2 sour apples

2 mugs rosemary tea

Lunch

- 1 cup of any of the following beans in any combination:
  Adzuki, black, great northern, pinto
- 2 cups of any of the following, steamed:
  Asparagus, broccoli, cabbage, endive, escarole, parsley, scallion, spinach, summer squash, zucchini
- Repeat breakfast supplement recommendations.

Midafternoon Snack

- Repeat breakfast smoothie but omit supplements.

Dinner

- Repeat lunch and breakfast supplements.

Evening

2 mugs rosemary tea

The WHD Five-Day Metabolic Detox Diet and Supplement Plan is designed to cleanse the body of free-radical by-products, heavy metals, potentially harmful fat-soluble compounds, toxic hormones, allergens, and acute inflammatory agents.

Now that your metabolism has been given every imaginable advantage to function at its highest possible level, you're ready to move on to the WHD nutrition primer.

Stimulating Metabolism with Physical Exercise

Let's make one important point right off the bat. Studies have clearly shown that successful weight loss can be attained by following a program of proper dieting without exercise. While scientifically factual, this sends a bad message. Nature intended our bodies to engage in movement, endurance, strength building, balance, and flexibility. Each of us is the natural genetic by-product of millions of years of running, jumping, climbing, and swimming. Physical exercise is vital to our overall health and metabolic function. A strong body is vital to our holistic balance.

There are four major types of physical exercise: endurance, strength, balance, and flexibility.

Endurance exercise includes running, jogging, brisk walking, hiking, biking, and rowing. Yard work in virtually any capacity also increases the heart rate.

Strength exercise includes weight lifting, Nautilus training, resistance band exercises, and nearly any form of physical activity that increases the delivery of oxygen and blood to muscles.

Balance and flexibility exercise includes martial arts, tai chi, qigong, and yoga.

Where the mantra of the Whole Health Diet program is balance, it is advised that one engage in a combination of all the aforementioned exercises. That said, there are a few key points regarding exercise that are of great importance to the issue of weight loss.

One common misconception about metabolism is that by simply engaging in vigorous aerobic exercise, our bodies will burn the maximum amount of calories. Every time I go to the gym, I see overweight exercisers on treadmills determined to sweat off the pounds. Though they're clearly well intentioned, the concept of muscle building for the purposes of boosting metabolism and burning calories seems to elude them. By increasing heart rate with aerobic exercise, one will absolutely increase metabolism, but only in the short term. Weight training and muscle building will burn fewer calories in the short term, but it's been shown to increase metabolic efficiency and calorie-burning output in the long term. Each pound of muscle burns 40 calories per day, while each pound of fat burns only 2 calories. Increased muscle mass means you can consume more food and gain less weight. Much more about food later, but for now the important point is if you want to support your metabolism in the most efficient manner, it's important that you make a commitment to a balanced exercise program.

The WHD program recommends alternating forty-minute sessions of aerobic exercise, thirty-minute sessions of weight/resistance training, and some form of mind-body exercise (tai chi, yoga, martial arts) as your schedule allows.

CHAPTER 4

THE WHOLE HEALTH DIET PRIMER

If You Want to Be Lean You Have to Eat Clean

This morning I had a consultation with a twenty-eight-year-old woman from the Ukraine, who told me that she'd gained twenty pounds over the course of a few short months. She attributed the sudden weight gain solely to her transition from Ukrainian to American food. She said that while living in the Ukraine, she ate exclusively farm-fresh, organic food. Though it may be hard to believe, our foods have been denatured, processed, and, in some cases, even toxically designed to increase their addictive potential. Experts now tell us that as many as 250 million Americans are addicted to artificial food chemicals. Simply stated, food is a drug. Drugs can save lives, and drugs can take lives. Moreover, the dangerous drugs that are our most toxic foods are destroying our metabolisms and contributing mightily to the overweight and obesity epidemic.

All foods fall into one of three categories: toxic, neutral, or medicinal.

Whether your nutritional goal is to beat cancer or lose weight, the quality of your food must be medicinal. When it comes specifically to weight loss, the energetic properties of food exert a powerful influence on rate of metabolism. The WHD emphasizes that in order for your diet to be healthy, holistic, and metabolically balanced, it must comprise only the most healthy, nontoxic, and anti-inflammatory foods. This can be a tall order.

Today, our foods are chemically and biologically engineered beyond recognition. Concerned only about minimizing their losses and maximizing their sales, the commercial "food factories" are hell-bent on preserving, texturizing, flavor enhancing, coloring, and conditioning our foods. In all, the FDA now permits over eighty thousand chemicals to be added to American food. Furthermore, our foods are in serious trouble long before they ever reach the marketplace. The problem begins with the ravaged soil in which our food is grown. Experts estimate that due to depleted farming soil, our produce is now losing as much as 10 percent of its nutrient value every decade.

Until the mid-1940s, American farmers returned vital nutrients to the soil by age-old means of mulching, crop rotation, and manuring. All of these methods represent successful means of enriching soil, and thus foods' nutrient quality, employed since the beginning of time. By the end of the Second World War, drug conglomerates had stockpiled vast amounts of nitrates and phosphates, originally manufactured for weapons development. Hard-pressed to find markets for these leftover chemical compounds, many of these companies turned to the agricultural industry to sell their wares. Experiments at that time had proven that crops would thrive on a blend of nitrogen, potassium, and phosphorus. Armed with this information, war chemicals manufacturers descended upon the farm industry of America with nitrate-phosphate fertilizers at attractive, dramatically reduced costs. By the early 1960s, the American farm industry had become totally converted to synthetic fertilizing. Today, the sad realities of chemical fertilizing, hybridizing, and quick growing time continue to deplete our foods of their nutrients long before they leave the farm. Once they reach the marketplace, our foods are then assaulted by food manufacturers who proceed to cold store, dry, salt, pickle, sugar, ferment, smoke, freeze, can, preserve, artificially enrich, and irradiate them. Studies show that such treatment accounts for nutrient loss reaching levels of up to 80 percent.

Far worse than the nutrient depletion of our foods, manufacturers are now poisoning our foods with dangerous toxic chemicals. Among the stockpile of chemicals added to our foods today are dyes, bleaches, emulsifiers, antioxidants, preservatives, flavor enhancers, buffers, sprays, acidifiers, alkalizers, deodorants, gases, drying agents, curers, fortifiers, hydrolyzers, antifoaming agents, anticaking agents, and hydrogenators. One Surgeon General's Report on Nutrition and Health estimated that as many as ten thousand cancer deaths per year were very possibly due to food additives.[1] This is especially disconcerting when you consider that recent studies show that the average American consumes approximately 140 to 150 pounds of food additives per year.[2] It's a dark and dismal picture.

Our foods are fatted, sugared, and even genetically modified. Ninety percent of our produce is grown on synthetic fertilizers, injected with growth hormones, sprayed with inordinate concentrations of deadly pesticides, doused with antibiotics, or even DNA altered. According to the organization Healthy

Child Healthy World, 70 percent of the total calories consumed by Americans come from highly processed foods—a fivefold increase since the 1950s. They tell us that the average American child consumes more than five servings of pesticides and 150 mg of artificial food coloring every day.[3] These disturbing facts about the deteriorating state of American food are clearly getting the attention of the whole world. Up to 80 percent of the prepackaged foods on our grocery shelves are banned in most other countries. In fact, there are currently fifty countries in the world that refuse to import American food—and there are only 196 countries in the world today. The website GlobalResearch.ca recently highlighted a story that exemplifies just how poorly the world now views the deteriorating and toxic quality of American food:

"It's sad when one of the biggest 'super powers' can't even export a quintessentially American food to another country because it is too toxic to eat. But apples treated with diphenylamine (DPA), a substance which keeps them from turning brown for months at a time when they are kept in storage, is now a sore spot for importers of American apples.

"DPA isn't harmful all by itself, but it breaks down into carcinogenic elements. It's been used since 1962, but was banned in the European Union in 2012 since producers couldn't answer inquiries about its safety. European food safety regulators wanted more information on it, but none could be summoned. The apple industry simply responded with one study 'that detected three unknown chemicals on DPA-treated apples, but it could not determine if any of these chemicals, apparently formed when the DPA broke down, were nitrosamines.'

"British scientists, John Barnes and Peter Magee, in 1956, reported that dimethylnitrosamine produced liver tumors in rats, and later went on to test other nitrosamines and N-nitroso compounds. They found that the compounds caused all kinds of problems, including liver cancer, lung cancer, and even botulism."[4]

Many of our foods also contain known carcinogenic (cancer-causing) chemicals such as bisphenol A, bromates, phthalates, bovine growth hormone, and vinyl chloride. The efficiency of our general chemistry, including our metabolic calorie-burning chemistry, is dependent upon the efficiency of the chemistry in our foods. In simple terms, a machine is only as good as its fuel. In order to support our miracle machine's efficient burning of calories, we must first ensure that the fuel we feed it is of the highest nature.

The WHD emphasizes that all foods are classified as either toxic, neutral, or medicinal. One of the most important first steps of the WHD journey is to eliminate toxic foods, reduce neutral foods, and increase the more beneficial medicinal foods. To keep things simple, there are four major classifications of toxic foods:

1. POISONOUS FOODS:
Any food that is not classified as USDA organic, free range, and wild

2. JUNK FOODS:
Processed sugars and high-sugar products (including candies, cakes, pies, cookies, ice cream, and soft drinks)
Processed, high-starch products (including crackers, pretzels, and chips)
Fried foods

White flour

White rice

Fast food (including commercial hamburgers, hot dogs, and pizza)

Juices

High-fat foods (including cream soups, condiments, gravies, cream
    sauces, and toppings)

3. FERMENTED FOODS. Before going on to the fermented food list, we should
have a brief discussion about fermented foods. At present, many people are
encouraging the use of fermented foods, pointing to their well-noted health
claims. Advocates note that fermented foods, because of their ability to produce an abundance of healthy, living enzymes and beneficial bacteria in the
body, were a natural part of our ancestors' diets and supported their health
and longevity. I feel it's very important to understand that all foods have dual
properties. That is, every food under the sun is representative of both yin
and yang simultaneously. By this I mean that every food—not unlike every
person and every other dynamic living thing in the world—possesses the
potential to produce both good and bad results. The downside of fermented
foods is that they can, in some cases, increase bloating, gas, single-cell bacteria buildup in the intestines, and yeast infections. It depends upon who's
consuming them. The WHD emphasizes that, unlike us, our ancestors
weren't weaned on high concentrations of sugar, yeasted bread, pizza, baked
goods, marinades, condiments, processed vinegars, beer, wine, and champagne. Therefore, their ability to tolerate limited amounts of "natural" fermentation was far greater than ours today. Their bodies, much cleaner than

ours, were better able to benefit from the positive, healthy aspects of clean fermentation.

I can't tell you how many people I've worked with over the years who lost incredible amounts of weight, but still looked like they were overweight because of bloating around the midsection from too much fermentation in the gut. When you work that hard to lose weight, you shouldn't have to contend with what I call "belly puff." So let's take a look at the fermented-food list:

Yeasted breads

Mushrooms, morels, truffles

Vinegars and marinades

Nuts and seeds

Melons

Beer, wine, and champagne

Fermented soy (including miso, tempeh, tamari, and soy sauce)

Aged cheeses (especially blue, Limburger, cheddar, Parmesan, and Asiago)

People are often confused by this list of fermented foods to avoid. Melons themselves are not fermented, but because they contain such a high concentration of water and are grown so close to the ground, they're inclined to produce mold. Consuming an abundance of high-mold foods increases one's likelihood of intestinal bloat from fungal proliferation in the intestines.

4. INFLAMMATORY FOODS. It's important to keep in mind that the word "inflammation" no longer merely refers to achy joints. We now know that inflammation refers to a process in which dietary fats from foods are trans-

formed into bad eicosanoids—hormones capable of turning on disease gene switches. Many experts now believe that inflammation is responsible for nearly 75 percent of all diseases, including type 2 diabetes and obesity. The most important point regarding inflammatory foods and weight loss is that inflammatory foods drive up the ratio of bad to good eicosanoids in the body. This dramatically increases the likelihood of fat storage. Let's have a look at the inflammatory foods list:

Food allergens
Red meats
Dairy products
Egg yolks
Nuts, especially peanuts (but see note below)
Nori seaweed
Tilapia
Catfish
Duck
Fried foods
Yellowtail
Most vegetable oils (except for olive and flaxseed)
Processed sugars and high starches

Let's take a minute to clear up any confusion regarding nuts, such as almonds and walnuts, which are generally not listed as inflammatory. Almonds are typically categorized as a neutral food, while walnuts are considered anti-inflammatory. Following the lead of *Whole Health*, the WHD underscores the point that because fat represents the most vital nutrient in nuts, nature places them in a protective shell. The shell protects the prized, nutrient-rich fats in nuts from heat and moisture. Overexposure to high heat makes fats susceptible to potentially disease-causing free-radical peroxides, and moisture makes them susceptible to a mutation-triggering single-cell fungus. Thus, by removing the shells from nuts to make them more consumer friendly, the food industry is unwittingly increasing their inflammatory potential. So as you can see, once exposed to heat and/or moisture, anti-inflammatory nuts like walnuts can go from anti-inflammatory to inflammatory.

Do Not Trust the Food Industry!

Even as I write this, the food industry is feverishly at work trying to find new ways to hijack our brain chemistry and program us for addiction. Companies now employ an army of chemists, physicists, and neuroscientists who are contracted for the express purpose of engineering their foods to have the capability of stimulating our brain's reward center (nucleus accumbens), to ensure that we keep going back for more. They're researching ways to create the perfect blend of salt, sugar, fat, and additives to produce negative changes in heart rate and blood pressure that can only be stabilized by eating more. Most processed foods are now being flavored, textured, shaped, and sized to affect our brain's pleasure centers. This futuristic science has given rise to a whole new lexicon, as they evaluate foods for "mouth feel," "maximum bite force," "sensory specific satiety," and "the art of more-ish-ness." Their ultimate goal is to help us reach what they call "the bliss point." The industry now salaams to the mantra that "satiety is the enemy of food products."

Former industry executive Bruce Bradley, who spent fifteen years at General Mills, Pillsbury, and Nabisco working with some of the world's top scientists, one day discovered that he simply couldn't do it anymore. He has openly admitted that there were times he felt uncomfortable and troubled by what he was doing. He started to think about the products he was developing and how consumers were being chemically manipulated by them. He began to feel guilty about how his work was likely contributing to rising obesity trends and health problems. He now writes a blog critical of the food industry.

Make no mistake about it: they are now fully committed to proliferating generations of addicted consumers. Once they have us hooked, the mere sight of their product packaging will trigger our cravings. The food industry clearly has no conscience. Its chicanery is destined to dramatically increase the rate of food addiction in this country. We know beyond a shadow of a doubt that addictive overeating contributes mightily to obesity, which leads to heart disease and diabetes, which ultimately lead to untimely death. Any way you look at it, the food industry is getting away with murder.

Avoid Nonorganic Foods

We've all had those moments in life that we won't soon forget. I experienced one such occasion with my entire family many years ago. We'd just enjoyed a glorious family day at the beach, and we were all preparing dinner together in the kitchen. While dicing up bell peppers, my wife decided to take a little nibble. Within ten seconds of ingesting a small chunk of bell pepper, her throat began to close up. The entire family panicked, and what was a nice moment together had suddenly become an alarming experience. Fortunately, the ambulance arrived in the nick of time. She was attended to and stabilized within a matter of minutes. The cause of all this life-threatening mayhem was toxic pesticide exposure. This experience was a lesson for us all. It is truly astounding to think that such an innocent moment could be swiftly turned into a tragedy because of potentially life-threatening chemicals added to food.

I'm continually amazed at the number of patients I meet with who are still not completely sold on the idea of eating organic. Most point to the added expense, when they should be looking at the negative health potentials of eating nonorganic. Not only do nonorganic foods pose a threat to the immune system, but mounting research confirms that they may impair metabolism as well.

Most nonorganic foods are toxically laden with pesticides like malathion, diazinon, parathion, and chlorpyrifos. These pesticides are now referred to as obesogens. The term "obesogen" refers to an endocrine-disrupting chemical, or EDC, that leads to weight gain—and weight-gain-related diseases. They are also commonly found in food packaging plastics and additives. These obesogens mimic human hormones by disrupting the programming of stem cells so that they become fat cells, and by altering natural gene function. In so doing, they create severe glandular imbalances, disrupting the body's ability to regulate weight. In short, obesogenic pesticides common to nonorganic foods make us fat.

Every day, the average American is exposed to up to thirteen pesticides. Researchers at the University of California, Irvine, have found that animals exposed to pesticides tend to have higher levels of fat cell formation and are generally more likely to gain weight later in life. The research team believes the same holds true for humans.[5] Similarly, a recent human study showed that the adult daughters of women who were exposed to the highest levels of DDT during their childbearing years were found to be twenty pounds heavier on average than the daughters of women who had the lowest exposure levels.[6] The causal connection to all this weight-gain-causing endocrine disruption appears to be thyroid deficiency.

As covered on nbcnews.com, "Researchers have noted a link between organochlorine pesticides and impaired thyroid function. According to the Endocrine Society's 2009 report on EDCs, changes in thyroid function can result in metabolic effects. Indeed, the authors of a 2009 *Thyroid Research* article cited hypothyroidism, a symptom of which can be weight gain, as a possible effect of organochlorines on the thyroid.

"The authors of a study in the journal *BioScience* found that tributyltin, a fungicide, activates components in human cells known as retinoid X receptors, which are part of the metabolic pathway necessary for fat-cell formation. They also found that tributyltin causes the growth of fat cells in mice exposed to it. Although tributyltin is no longer used on crops, experts suspect that a similar compound still used on produce, called fenbutatin, is at least as potent.

"The authors of a recent study in *Molecular and Cellular Endocrinology* note that organophosphates and carbamates, two common classes of pesticides, cause obesity in animals."[7]

One recent study published in the *American Journal of Epidemiology* established a connection between an increased risk of thyroid disease and exposure to pesticides among women. The study looked at North Carolina and Iowa women who were married to men who routinely used pesticides like aldrin, DDT, and lindane in their work. The researchers found that these women were at a significantly higher risk of developing thyroid conditions than were women in non-agricultural areas. Of the 16,500 wives studied, over 12 percent were ultimately diagnosed with thyroid disease, compared to between 1 and 8 percent of the population at large.[8] The nonprofit group Beyond Pesticides reports that some 60 percent of the pesticides commonly in use today have been shown to affect the human thyroid gland's production of T_3 and T_4 hormones.[9]

The good news is that experts say we can reduce our pesticide exposure by nearly 80 percent simply by choosing organic versions of the twelve fruits and vegetables shown in tests to contain the highest pesticide load. The nonprofit Environmental Working Group has termed them the Dirty Dozen. In order of highest to lowest pesticide load, they are: apples, peaches, nectarines, strawberries, grapes, celery, spinach, sweet bell peppers, cucumbers, cherry tomatoes, snap peas, and potatoes. The group also lists what they call the Clean Fifteen, those conventionally grown fruits and vegetables with the lowest pesticide residue: avocados, sweet corn, pineapples, cabbage, sweet peas, onions, asparagus, mangoes, papayas, kiwi, eggplant, grapefruit, cantaloupe, cauliflower, and sweet potatoes.[10]

Detoxify Your Produce

One antidote to all this toxic pesticide exposure is to become a better label reader and to purchase only USDA organic food. If you feel you can't afford organic foods or if for some reason you don't have access, the WHD offers a simple, helpful solution. Purchase two sixteen-ounce spray bottles from your neighborhood hardware store and fill each with fifteen ounces of tap water. In one bottle, add one teaspoon of apple cider vinegar, and in the other bottle add one teaspoon of baking soda. Label them both and keep them readily available. Next, a natural bristle brush and a colander are needed. Simply spray produce first with the cider vinegar solution and follow that with the baking soda solution. Finally, brush the produce briskly, place in the colander, and rinse with cold tap water. This simple procedure will both cleanse and neutralize many of the insecticide residues and poisons that coat your fresh produce. Even though there are a number of other methods, I've always found this one to be the simplest and most convenient.

Avoid Genetically Modified Foods

Like many, I am of the belief that food is medicine. I can remember back to the 1976 McGovern Senate subcommittee's groundbreaking diet and human needs findings. After having heard testimony from 1,100 of the world's most respected doctors and researchers from eight different countries, the subcommittee stated in its findings that we could prevent 30 percent of all cancer, heart disease, and diabetes-related deaths with diet alone. This was the first government-organized, taxpayer-funded program that clearly established that nutrition is indeed a viable form of preventive medicine.

Nowadays, millions of Americans are eating more fruits and vegetables and low-fat soy products to improve their health and prevent disease, but most of us do not fully understand the complexities of such a task. The food you're eating today is not your grandmother's food. In fact, most of what you're eating has been genetically altered.

Genetically modified organisms (GMOs) and genetically engineered organisms (GEOs) are those whose genetic material has been altered using genetic engineering techniques. These techniques—generally known as "recombinant DNA technology"—use DNA from different sources that are combined into one molecule to create a new set of genes. This newly formed DNA is then transferred into living organisms, providing them with a modified genetic structure. In short, this is an experiment in manipulating DNA to create novel proteins. To most, this would seem like an exercise fraught with peril, but proponents have a different view.

The world population is over seven billion, and it's predicted to increase by 50 percent over the next fifty years. GMO advocates, like the Monsanto Company, insist that the genetic engineering of food will ensure an adequate food supply for the world's booming population. They also underscore the GMO benefits of pest resistance, herbicide tolerance, disease resistance, freeze tolerance, and drought tolerance. While the technology of genetic modification has its advocates, many people are gravely concerned about the potential of human health risks. Questions have been raised about cancer, allergies, unknown immune effects, and ecological oversight.

The Monsanto Company is a U.S.-based, multinational, agricultural biotechnology corporation. It is the leading producer of genetically engineered seeds and provides the technology for 90 percent of the world's GEO seeds. Over the past three decades Monsanto has been on a fast track to genetically modify and patent the world's crops. The company first announced its intentions to insert genetically modified organisms from viruses, bacteria, insects, animals, and even humans into the DNA of crops and animals in 1983. Monsanto is also positioning itself to buy up all the world's available heirloom seeds with the aim of controlling the world's food supply.

Currently, 90 percent of our soy, 88 percent of our corn, and 80 percent of all processed foods on our supermarket shelves are genetically modified. According to the U.S. Department of Agriculture, there are over forty plant varieties for which companies have fulfilled federal requirements for genetic commercialization. Monsanto is not alone in this exploit. Its vision is shared by many other companies, large and small, worldwide. A company from Massachusetts called AquaBounty is presently working on genetically modifying salmon to speed up the growth cycle in order to get it to market faster.

Proponents of this technology are often quick to point out that only nine foods are currently being genetically modified full scale: soy, corn, cottonseed oil, canola oil, sugar beets, Hawaiian papaya, alfalfa, zucchini, and summer squash. However, truth be told, genetic modification is seeping into our food supply by an array of other means.

Many of us are being exposed to GMOs via dairy, beef, poultry, and pork livestock feed. Most of our food additives, flavor enhancers, excipients (bulking agents), binders, and fillers are also genetically modified. As if that's not enough, many of our alcoholic beverages, baked goods, and juices are also genetically modified. Perhaps most disappointing of all, 99 percent of vitamin C and most of our vitamin E in virtually all of our gel-coated vitamins are now genetically modified. Big Pharma's also gotten into the act. In 2012, the FDA approved the first GMO prescription medicine, Elelyso, which was developed to treat an enzyme deficiency condition called Gaucher. The replacement enzymes provided by Elelyso are derived from GMO carrots. There are a host of other GMO pharmaceuticals about to appear on the scene. The scientific journal *Nature* recently published a report on a study published in the *Journal of the American Medical Association* stating that GMO medicines, or "biologicals," are potentially twice as dangerous as the average pharmaceutical drug.[11] This is especially disturbing when you consider that currently, one hundred thousand Americans are killed and three million are hospitalized because of the negative side effects of prescription drugs each year. Genetic modification is becoming insidious in our foods, as it's showing up just about everywhere.

Monsanto's genetically engineered bovine growth hormone (rBGH, also called rBST) is being injected into cows in order to increase milk production. Milk from those cows treated with growth hormone contains significantly higher levels (up to ten times) of a hormone called insulin-like growth factor (IGF-1). IGF-1 has been linked to a sevenfold increased risk for breast cancer among premenopausal women under the age of fifty and a fourfold increased risk for prostate cancer among men, as well as generally increased risks for colon and lung cancers.[12]

A number of other studies have demonstrated that GMOs may pose serious risks of toxicity, allergenicity, antibiotic resistance, immunosuppression, environmental pollution, and genetic contamination. The first long-term study of the effects of GMOs, performed at the University of Caen in France, found that genetically modified foods consistently caused large tumors in animals. Additional French studies discovered that three varieties of Monsanto GMO corn were linked to kidney and liver damage in rats.[13] A 2009 Russian study linked GMO soy to sterility, birth defects, and growth and reproduction problems in animals.[14] Over the past thirty years, I've counseled tens of thousands of patients, many with serious health conditions rooted in serious food allergies. Once a patient identifies and avoids using an allergenic food, his or her health generally tends to improve significantly. I've seen patients diagnosed with serious diseases who went on to experience complete recovery—and the first step was discontinuing their use of toxic, allergenic foods. Now with so many unlabeled GMO foods in play, the whole game's been changed.

The industry is genetically inserting such a wide variety of foods and organisms into so many of the foods we eat, without labeling, that it's becoming virtually impossible to avoid potential symptoms. Suppose, for example, you're allergic to a specific species of North Atlantic fish. Over millennia, that fish has developed genes that protect it from freezing to death in frigid waters. The GMO food industry might well be attracted to the prospect of isolating the "antifreeze" genes from that fish, for the purposes of inserting them into something like strawberries to protect them from freeze damage. This may be great for the grower, but not for you. You eat the strawberries and before long you're on your way to the emergency room. Moreover, the ER doctors will never know what's causing your inflammatory, anaphylactic reaction, because there was no labeling on the cross-contaminated berries you just ate.

To date, Congress has not passed any legislation to protect you, the consumer, and your family from such potential disaster, and the FDA has imposed no safety testing requirements. When it comes to GMO technology, there is not a single safety standard required of the food industry. According to a recent national poll, 91 percent of the American public don't want to eat genetically modified food. The problem is, there are no guidelines in place to assist consumers in their attempts to avoid purchasing GMO foods.

The agribusiness industry continues to push against the idea of voluntary GMO labeling. It supports a more free market approach to product labeling. Consumer groups, however, believe that people simply have the right to know. They support efforts for a mandatory labeling plan.

Currently, the FDA's outdated position on GMO labeling is governed by the Food, Drug, and Cosmetic Act, which contends only with food additives. The FDA takes the position that there is no appreciable difference between GMO and non-GMO foods. In order for foods to be labeled as GMO and non-GMO, Congress would be forced to engage in a behemoth bureaucratic effort that would demand sweeping changes in the present food labeling policy. There are also important questions regarding how to determine acceptable limits as well as effective detection.

That said, every consumer should know these all-important guidelines. Don't count on any "All Natural" labels; they offer the consumer virtually no protection whatsoever! Also, don't count on the "Made with Organic Ingredients" label. This label indicates only that the food in question is required to be 70 percent organic. The "Contains Organic Ingredients" label means exactly the same thing. Look for the USDA Organic seal. Only foods that are 95 to 100 percent organic and GMO-free can bear this label.

There are also important environmental questions that must be answered. Environmental activists, public interest groups, religious organizations, and green lobbies have all raised concerns regarding GMO agribusiness from the standpoint of potential hazardous toxins, environmental concerns, and conservational risks. There have been a number of studies that have correlated insect and other species extinction with GMO technology. Most noteworthy here is the recent controversial research that implicates GMO corn pollen in monarch butterfly/caterpillar extinction.

The problem of gene transfer to nontarget species is also of growing concern. Crops engineered for herbicide tolerance have interbred with weeds, resulting in "superweeds" that have drawn a good deal of recent legal attention in a rash of newly filed farmer lawsuits against Monsanto. While the farmers cry foul about the cross-pollination nightmare, Monsanto has gone on the offensive, claiming that these farmers have obtained Monsanto-licensed seeds from an unknown source, for which it claims they have failed to pay royalties. The GMO wars rage on.

Regardless of your position on GMO foods, there should be no doubt that the consumer deserves to be better supported by a government that claims to be "for the people." We the people deserve to be better informed with proper GMO labeling. Let the buyer beware, but first arm buyers with the facts as to exactly what they are purchasing. If GMO is a consumer-safe technology, then there should be nothing to hide.

According to a number of recent studies, genetically modified foods may contribute to weight gain and obesity. A recent comparative analysis of animal blood and organ systems data showed that rats that were fed GMO corn experienced an increase in overall body weight of about 3.7 percent, with an increase in liver weight of approximately 11 percent.[15] In another study, Norwegian researchers fed one group of rats genetically modified corn while another group was fed GMO-free corn. After only ninety days, the rats that were fed the GMO corn grew much fatter and developed much bigger appetites than the non-GMO-fed rats. The researchers repeated the same experiment, but they replaced the rats with mice, fish, and snakes, and were surprised to find that they ended up with the exact same results.[16] Researchers from the nations of Austria, Hungary, Ireland, Turkey, and Australia participated in the study, while the United States was not represented.

The WHD emphasizes the point that a number of studies continue to demonstrate that GMO foods are linked to weight gain and obesity. Consider the fact that nutrition is a biochemical game of pitch and catch. Whenever we eat, foods and nutrients are "pitched" into our bodies. We have chemical receptors and enzymes that will then "catch," or absorb and assimilate them. Common sense suggests that those little nutrient "catcher's mitts" in our bodies were designed from millions of years of genetic evolution, and that over that period of time they became accustomed to catching the same foods and nutrients as have always been provided by nature. Suddenly, out of the blue, they're being asked to recognize and catch something that they've never seen before. Now the foods and nutrients they have to contend with have undergone such a genetic makeover, the old game of pitch and catch has likely been changed forever. And if our bodies cannot recognize, absorb, and assimilate foods, then they are more likely to simply store them. Also, it's not just a case of weight gain caused by genetic confusion. It's also a case of poor food generally meaning more food.

According to a recent landmark study, researchers from the University of Texas at Austin studied U.S. Department of Agriculture nutritional data on forty-three different vegetables and fruits and found reliable declines in the amount of protein, calcium, phosphorus, iron, vitamin B2, and vitamin C over the past half century.[17] This is believed to be due to the fact that genetically modified crops are being bred for higher yields. The more food we are pressed to produce within shorter windows of time, the less efficient or lower the nutrient concentrations. The lower the nutrient concentrations, the more our bodies have to consume in order to make up the difference. If you wish to keep your calorie count from going up, you'll have to put the GMO foods down!

Avoid High-Fructose Corn Syrup

The current processing of our food is creating metabolic mayhem. It's becoming very clear that our overweight and obesity epidemic is directly related to our toxic food. Most of our processed foods today contain high concentrations of bioengineered high-fructose corn syrup (HFCS), a proven metabolic saboteur. Composed of over 50 percent fructose, HFCS is said to be over 70 percent hidden from us—that is to say, it's been given a variety of different chemical names to hide behind. So, when reading food labels, if you see names like maize syrup, glucose syrup, glucose/fructose syrup, tapioca syrup, roasted dahlia syrup, fruit fructose, or crystalline fructose, then run the other way! Many experts estimate that the average American today consumes up to sixty pounds of HFCS per year. Not so coincidentally, since HFCS first appeared in the standard American diet, obesity rates have tripled and diabetes has increased sevenfold. The primary reason for its likely contribution is that high-fructose corn syrup contains free-form monosaccharides of fructose and glucose, which represent a fructose-glucose bond that dramatically slows its metabolic breakdown in the body. This means a nightmare weight loss metabolism. Fructose is delivered directly to the liver. The high concentrations of this poorly assimilated sugar ultimately sabotage the liver's efforts to perform the all-important function of anaerobic glycolysis, resulting in a slowing down of metabolism and a higher rate of fat storage.

According to a study published online in February 2010 in the journal *Pharmacology, Biochemistry and Behavior*, a Princeton University research team demonstrated that rats with access to high-fructose corn syrup gained significantly more weight than counterparts who were given access to table sugar. Both groups consumed the same amount of total calories. The researchers also noted that the rats fed high-fructose corn syrup also experienced highly abnormal increases in body fat, especially around the abdomen, from high concentrations of circulating triglyceride blood fats. One of the researchers, Bart Hoebel, who is a psychology professor and a specialist in the neuroscience of appetite, weight, and sugar addiction, went on to say, "Some people have claimed that high-fructose corn syrup is no different than other sweeteners when it comes to weight gain and obesity, but our results make it clear that this just isn't true, at least under the conditions of our tests. When rats are drinking high-fructose corn syrup at levels well below those in soda pop, they're becoming obese— every single one, across the board. Even when rats are fed a high-fat diet, you don't see this; they don't all gain extra weight."[18] A second study was conducted by the same research team and similar results were found. The animals who were given access to high-fructose corn syrup gained 48 percent more weight than those eating a diet free of the substance.

Avoid Trans Fat

When it comes to dietary needs, there is no fat that poses a greater threat to our health than trans fat, or trans-fatty acids (TFAs). Trans fat has been shown to raise bad cholesterol and lower good cholesterol. This deadly combination dramatically increases the risk of heart disease. TFAs are produced through a process called hydrogenation, in which hydrogen molecules are added to vegetable oils to extend their shelf life. Once again, the food industry has found a way to protect its investment at the cost of our health. The extra hydrogen molecule that's added to these fats may prevent spoilage, but it also has a way of confusing the human body, which is unable to detect the unnatural molecule, as it's only designed to recognize natural fats. Thus, the body doesn't fully break down these processed fats, which then remain stuck in the arteries and all around the heart. Unfortunately, most of the foods that are highest in TFAs tend to be favorite kid foods. Among those foods highest in TFAs are cookies, cakes, pies, crackers, doughnuts, and french fries. And if you think you're safe by reading labels, guess again. For example, if a food contains less than 0.5 grams of trans fat per serving, the food label is legally permitted to read "0 g." Thus, if a person were to consume multiple servings of products that are said to contain zero grams of trans fat, he or she could still actually exceed safe recommended limits. The key when reading labels is to search for the term "partially hydrogenated vegetable oil." This is the only way to identify the presence of trans fat in a product. The word "partially" is very important. Avoid foods that contain partially hydrogenated oils. This might seem a little confusing, but if the label reads "fully" or "completely" hydrogenated oil, it doesn't contain trans fat.

Avoid Toxic BPA Plastics

Many of our drinking water bottles and leftover food storage containers are made of plastics that contain bisphenol A (BPA). The National Institute of Environmental Health Sciences considers BPA research a high priority because of its demonstrated potential for adverse effects. BPA is a toxic faux estrogen and an endocrine disrupter, and a number of animal and human cross-sectional studies have shown that it increases appetite, slows metabolism, causes weight gain, and contributes to insulin resistance, thyroid dysfunction, and obesity. The WHD advises that you replace all your plastic, carbon-based drinking water bottles and food storage containers with glass, ceramic, and stainless steel alternatives. Klean Kanteen water bottles are among the best options for the safe, affordable storage of your drinking water. An 18 ounce bottle is generally priced at around twenty dollars.

The WHD Nutrition Primer
(Clean and Healthy Eating)

Now that your pantry, cabinets, refrigerator, and freezer are all safe and clean, we can get ready to move on to the WHD basic diet design, but just before we do, we'll need to get our nutritional bearings with the WHD primer.

Proteins. The word "protein" comes from the Greek word for "primary." I often refer to proteins as the body's department of public works, because their primary responsibility is to build, regulate, and repair. As we repair, we offset aging. Therefore, quality dietary proteins are essential for longevity. As dermatologist Nicholas Perricone writes, "The building blocks of our cells are composed of amino acids. As protein is digested, it breaks down into amino acids that are then used by the cells to repair themselves. Without adequate protein, our bodies enter into an accelerated aging mode. Our muscles, organs, bones, cartilage, skin, and the antibodies that guard us from disease are all made of protein. Even the enzymes that facilitate all-important chemical reactions, from digestion to building cells, are made of protein. This simple fact of life can change the way you look beginning with your next meal. If your cells do not have complete availability of all essential amino acids, cellular repair will not only be incomplete but also will be much slower than it should be."[19]

Proteins are made up of amino acids, catalysts that activate, direct, and energize cells. In all, there are twenty amino acids. The human body produces only eleven of them; therefore, nine amino acids that are considered essential for human health need to come from outside sources. The building block amino acids that make up proteins represent a primary reason why proteins burn calories and carbohydrates generate fat. A number of studies show that amino acids are essential for metabolic management and weight loss. Among the most important weight loss amino acids are L-tyrosine (which supports healthy thyroid function), L-phenylalanine (which helps the brain to regulate appetite), and L-carnitine (which mobilizes fats from a storing to a burning mode). A balanced intake of quality proteins is an essential component to a fit, healthy diet plan.

Carbohydrates. Whereas proteins are responsible for building and repairing, carbohydrates provide fuel. The rate at which different carbohydrates provide the body with fuel is very important when it comes to healthy eating. Carbohydrates provide the body with fuel in the form of sugar. Some provide immediate fuel, while others provide a gradual release. The quicker a carbohydrate releases fuel (sugar), the more the body is inclined to store the remainder as fat. The slower a carbohydrate releases fuel, the less the body is inclined to store fat.

According to a report in *Time*, "New research suggests that it's the overconsumption of carbohydrates, sugars, and sweeteners that is chiefly responsible for the epidemics of obesity and type 2 diabetes. Refined carbohydrates, like those in wheat bread, hidden sugar, low-fat crackers, and pasta, cause changes in our blood chemistry that encourage the body to store the calories as fat and intensify hunger, making it much more difficult to lose weight."[20] Dietary fat has been a focus of human health for nearly seventy years, but we've only recently implicated carbohydrates.

The world has long been convinced that fewer calories, less fat consumption, and more exercise are the three simple keys to weight loss and heart health. From the 1950s until the mid-1980s, thanks in large part to the research of army doctor Ancel Keys, saturated fat and cholesterol consumption had been tagged as the leading causes of weight gain, obesity, and heart disease. We now know that fat is not the demon. Nutritional science has since discovered that 80 percent of the cholesterol in the human body is manufactured by the liver, triggered by the body's production of insulin that results from sugar and processed starch consumption. The key message here is: if you want to lose weight and lower your risks for obesity, type 2 diabetes, and heart disease, you need to cautiously monitor your carbohydrate consumption.

The WHD reminds us that there are two types of carbohydrates: low starch and high starch. Low-starch carbohydrates are best represented by low-sugar vegetables like asparagus, broccoli, spinach, and zucchini. First of all, yes, vegetables are carbohydrates! But due to the fact that these carbohydrates are low in sugar, they don't tend to be stored as fat. High-starch carbohydrates, on the other hand, are stored as fat. High-starch carbs, such as carrots, potatoes, rice, pasta, cereals, and breads, contain a higher concentration of sugar than do low-starch carbs; therefore, they store as fat at a significantly higher rate. A diet that's low in fat but high in starch carbohydrates is a diet that's high in fat storage. So, the lesson with carbohydrates is that it's not just what's on the plate, it's what it converts to once it's in the body. This is important when it comes to fruits as well.

It seems the whole world is of the opinion that fruits can do no wrong. Rich in fiber, antioxidants, vitamins, and minerals, fruits generally appear to be perfect foods for superior nutrition. But, truth be told, some fruits are major contributors to weight gain, obesity, type 2 diabetes, and heart disease. Not unlike vegetables, fruits also fall into two categories: low-sugar and high-sugar fruits. Low-sugar fruits, like blackberries, strawberries, apples, peaches, and mangoes, contain only about six to eight grams of sugar per serving (¾ cup). Once again, as with low-starch vegetables, low-sugar fruits tend to be stored significantly less as fat. High-sugar fruits, like oranges, pineapples, pears, bananas, and raisins, on the other hand, store as fat at a much higher rate.

Fats. Dietary fats are a form of stored energy. Too much fat-energy storage leads to an overweight condition, obesity, and heart disease. Interestingly enough, it takes a certain amount of healthy fat to burn unwanted stored fats. There are good fats and there are bad fats. Saturated fat, trans fat, and rancid fat are among the unhealthiest of all food sources. Unhealthy, stored body fats are readily burned and converted into fuel within our cellular mitochondria, but only when healthy, essential fatty acids, or EFAs, are abundant in the body.

EFAs are considered essential because we cannot naturally synthesize them on our own. We can obtain them only from proper nutrition. Two of these fatty acids are considered essential for human health: alpha-linolenic acid (omega-3 fatty acid) and linoleic acid (omega-6 fatty acid). These two all-important essential fatty acids, often referred to as "vitamin F," form eicosanoid hormones that regulate immunity, inflammation, mood, behavior, and cell communication. In addition, essential fatty acids have been shown to suppress appetite and to increase metabolic function in the body by blocking genes that produce and store bad fats. Moreover, there is one form of essential omega-6 fatty acid naturally formed from a bacterium of meat and dairy products via an enzyme process called conjugated linoleic acid (CLA), which has been shown in a number of studies to help increase lean body mass while decreasing body fat.

One such study was a randomized, double-blind, placebo-controlled trial performed at the University of North Carolina and published in the *Journal of Nutrition*. This study found that supplementation with 6.4 grams of CLA per day for twelve weeks increased lean body mass among obese adult subjects.[21]

In another study, performed by the Scandinavian Clinical Research Group and published in the *American Journal of Clinical Nutrition*, CLA supplementation was proven to assist in lipid reduction, as one group of overweight women lost 9 percent of their body fat in one year.[22]

There is also an omega-7 monounsaturated fatty acid, called palmitoleic acid, that's often referred to as the "essential nonessential fatty acid." Omega-7 fatty acid may be found in freshwater fish, macadamia nuts, and sea buckthorn berries and is purported to have numerous skin and health benefits. Omega-7 fatty acids are best known for their unsurpassed support for cholesterol reduction and weight loss metabolism.

The WHD—Basic Design

It's important to mention that this section of the book is intended to present you with the *basic* WHD design. Chapter 6 provides all the details of the WHD's Electromagnetic Muscle Testing (EMT) and Acutrition systems, which will teach you how to customize your very own personalized diet, enabling you to fully maximize your metabolic and nutritional energies. Remember, as you read the following pages, that this is only the basic diet design. As you will clearly see in chapter 6, the WHD is the anti–one-size-fits-all plan.

Before outlining the basic design, it's important to keep in mind that the WHD is based on tens of thousands of successful private, corporate, and group weight loss consultations performed over the past three decades. And while there may be hundreds of weight loss theories and philosophies, few have been as successfully time-tested.

Please remember that all foods must be exclusively USDA organic, free range, and wild!

The WHD basic diet design might generally be described as a predominantly lean-protein, low-starch-vegetable, and low-sugar-fruit plan. The program is generally composed of three ¾-cup servings of protein, three ¾-cup servings of low-starch vegetables, two ½-cup servings of low-sugar fruit, one ¾-cup serving of high-starch carbohydrates, 3 tablespoons of monounsaturated oil, and 60 ounces of pure water per day.

Let's take a closer look at a sample day of general WHD eating:

BREAKFAST: Omelet (five egg whites) with ¾ cup low-starch vegetables; or a smoothie blend of two scoops of egg white protein (or brown rice protein powder), 10 ounces organic coconut milk, and ½ cup low-sugar fruit.

MIDMORNING: ½ cup berries, papaya, peaches, nectarines, and/or fresh apricots.

LUNCH: ½ cup poultry, wild fish, or organic beans with ¾ cup organic salad or low-starch vegetables. (If salad, dress with 2 tablespoons organic olive oil and lemon juice only.)

MIDAFTERNOON: Repeat midmorning snack.

DINNER: ½ cup wild fish, poultry, or beans, with ¾ cup low-starch vegetables, steamed.

EVENING: Try to avoid eating after dinner. Allow for twelve hours between the last bite of dinner and the first bite of breakfast.

WHOLE HEALTH DIETERS MAY CHOOSE FROM ANY ONE OF THE FOLLOW-ING STARCH OPTIONS TO EAT AT ANY ONE MEAL OF THE DAY: ¾ cup brown rice, brown rice pasta, quinoa, quinoa pasta, or baked white or sweet potato; or two slices of gluten-free, wheat-free, yeast-free bread.

LOW- TO MEDIUM-SUGAR FRUIT LIST: apples, fresh apricots, blackberries, blueberries, cranberries, grapefruit, guavas, raspberries, strawberries, papayas, peaches, and nectarines.

A NOTE ABOUT FRUITS: High-sugar fruits are four to six times higher in sugar than low-sugar fruits. High-sugar fruits convert to and store as fats more readily than low-sugar fruits.

FATS: 2 tablespoons of either extra-virgin olive oil, coconut oil, grape-seed oil, or flaxseed oil per day.

PREFERABLE SWEETENERS: 1 teaspoon of manuka honey or rice syrup, or 6 drops of liquid stevia per day.

SPICES: Basil, cinnamon, cumin, ginger, marjoram, oregano, parsley, rosemary, sage, thyme, and turmeric. (Limit the use of salt and pepper.)

A NOTE ABOUT SPICES: Researchers at the National Institute on Aging developed a unit of measurement for antioxidants called the ORAC value (for "oxygen radical absorbance capacity"). In 2006 researchers at the USDA used the ORAC factor as a means to evaluate hundreds of common foods and spices for their antioxidant values. Eight of the top ten highest-antioxidant foods were berries and beans. The single highest food was wild black raspberries, which totaled 19,671 ORAC points. Meanwhile ¼ teaspoon ground cloves totaled 290,283 points! The average serving of spice was ten to twenty times higher than the most antioxidant-rich foods. When it comes to building up your disease-preventing antioxidant factor, organic spices are equally, if not more, important than food and nutritional supplementation.

BEVERAGES: 60 ounces of pure water per day (distilled or reverse-osmosis treated, with maximum 50 ppm total dissolvable solids), coconut water, herb teas, freshly made juices, and/or coconut milk.

ADULT BEVERAGES: Unflavored top-shelf vodka (Chopin, Tito's) with effervescent mineral water and lime; tequila (Don Julio, Patrón). Do not exceed two drinks, two nights a week.

CHAPTER 5

A MATTER OF ENERGY

A Transformational Invitation

Whenever we view an object, our interpretation about what we're seeing is entirely dependent upon what we've been taught to believe we're looking at. I often reflect on a conversation I once had with a friend of mine from China. He explained to me that in his province in China, the intersections are governed completely differently than ours here in the West. He told me that the red lights and signs posted at the intersections indicate that the driver may proceed, while the green lights and signs direct them to stop. He told me that it was very difficult for him to reformat his mind for safe driving here in the United States.

I can relate. Having made some trips to Great Britain and Bermuda, I've often found myself feeling as though I was driving on the wrong side of the road, and even found myself drifting into the wrong lane from time to time. A programmed mind tends to see what it was programmed to *believe* it's looking at, rather than perceiving the truth of a situation.

Every culture is grounded in its own perceptions of reality, largely based on adopted systems and theories. Science, religion, and politics are among the many systems and theories that influence and shape our sociocultural beliefs. Once they're anchored, cultures embrace their sociocultural beliefs for generations. For example, for five thousand years, the East has commonly embraced the belief that qi, or life force energy, is the primary currency of life. The culture with the largest population on our planet has articulately developed a myriad of healing and self-defense systems based on this elusive concept. Chinese cultural reality is profoundly influenced by a history rich in mysticism and extrasensory perception. Here in the West, it's been a very different story. Our reality's been shaped by biological science and five-sensory perception. What we've always believed we were looking at has merely been a reflection of the matter we were taught to see.

As author Pam Grout explains in her book *E-Squared*, "Any illusionist worth his magic wand understands that the most important ingredient in his sleight-of-hand repertoire is diversion. A magician diverts his audience's attention *away* from what he's really doing and directs it *toward* something else that seems crucial but, of course, isn't.

"That's what we've done—diverted all our attention to the physical world. These sensory 'bluffs' have caused us to miss the fact that what is invisible, what we *can't* see with our eyes, is actually more fundamental to life than what we do see.

"Quantum physics tells us that the invisible energy realm—collectively referred to as the field, or the 'FP,' as I call it—is the primary governing force of the material realm. It's the blueprint that forms reality. Indeed, we now know the universe is made of nothing but waves and particles of energy that conform to our expectations, judgments, and beliefs.

"Subtle energies, thoughts, emotions, and consciousness play the starring roles in our life experiences, but because they're invisible, we haven't attempted to understand them or use them in our favor. To change the world is a simple matter of changing these expectations and beliefs. It's truly that easy. Bringing something into the physical world requires focusing not on what we see, but on what we *want* to see."[1]

The Western world long held fast to the belief that reality is a purely material proposition—humans are made of cells, chairs are made of wood, and cars are made of steel. Our perceptions, beliefs, and Newtonian illusions regarding a matter-based reality were firmly entrenched. Then, on November 9, 1922, when Albert Einstein was awarded the 1921 Nobel Prize in Physics for his work on the photoelectric effect, suddenly the game was changed. Einstein went on to further detail how energy creates matter, and that energy and matter are interconvertible and transferable.

All at once, our most fundamental governing concepts regarding our perceptions and beliefs about reality became obsolete. We learned from one of the most brilliant minds the world has ever known that humans are made up of more than cells, chairs are made up of more than wood, and cars are made up of more than steel. Suddenly we were forced to extend our thinking beyond our culture programming. We were now forced to consider a new reality, which asserted that life precedes cell, and it exists far beyond the five senses.

Einstein's work made it clear that the reality hierarchy doesn't begin with the cell, it begins with energy. Now we were compelled to acknowledge that material cells are made up of atoms, which in turn are composed of something that precedes them, called particles—particles of energy. In short, our view of reality, previously believed to be purely material, had been completely redefined as energy-established. Nonetheless, the biological science and five-sense perception that influenced our reality for so long has maintained an iron grip on our belief system.

I've often said that even though Einstein proved to us that energy creates matter, we've managed to resist surrendering our Newtonian ways for nearly a hundred years. We therefore should either take back his Nobel Prize or accept its transformational invitation.

It's natural for human beings to adapt, and equally natural for cultures to shift. Mass culture shifts are representative of large populations shedding their skin and evolving together as an extended family that's always in search of a better way to live. Culture shifts are about massive growth for the betterment of civilizations. Human beings are forced by nature to adapt and evolve in order to survive and to prosper. When any new idea comes along that offers to make life easier or better, the tribe generally gets on board. In fact the PC, the iPhone, and the ever-evolving world of apps are living proof that our tribe is ready, willing, and able to get on board. And while this is especially true regarding agents of material technology, it's also evident with energy.

It wasn't all that long ago when people in America, by and large, were unaware of yoga, tai chi, acupuncture, acupressure, qigong, and Reiki. I can remember when, not that many years ago, a vast majority of us thought of these energy-healing arts as nothing more than voodoo. Today, millions of Americans are routinely feeling their benefits.

It's becoming clear that something profound is happening in our world today. Global culture is, at present, transitioning radically. The world has at last caught up to Einstein, and the Internet has enticed us into its reality of unlimited information. It's a time of infinite possibility. Our thinking has radically changed and our consciousness has been infinitely expanded. We're both better equipped for and more in need of this radical change. Never before have human beings been so well informed. But, at the same time, never before have they been so overinformed. We've created a world that generates great intensity. The bombardment of information is accompanied by a deluge of expectation. Our nervous systems are being forced to operate on overload, and as they do, we have a greater need for a variety of systems that can render life support, healing, and stress relief. Where we, as a culture, once waited until we were ill to seek medical intervention, we're now inclined to employ health care support that enables us to prevent the onset of symptoms. So it's through this natural process of evolution and adaptation that we are suddenly finding it easier to open ourselves up to energy medicine. The present culture shift is reflecting a world that's gradually preparing to embrace the reality that everything is energy. Moreover, as we continue to evolve in our energy awareness we'll eventually come to understand that there is an infinite variety of energy applications that enable us to take our healing to a much higher level.

Energy

The first thing that comes to my mind whenever I hear the word "energy" is the dissimilarity of its Eastern and Western translations. Here in the West, "energy" is a noun that refers to the capacity to generate power or vigorous activity. Western science generally explains that energy manifests itself in four principal forms: potential energy, radiant energy, kinetic energy, and electromagnetic energy. For most of us mere mortals here in the modern West, the word "energy" refers to either what we don't have at four o'clock in the afternoon or what we hope we have enough of to heat and cool our homes. For our purposes in this book, "energy" refers to the animating force that vivifies all living things. Our use of the word will center on a more Eastern understanding.

In the East the word "energy" is synonymous with "life force." There are more than 150 words, in virtually every language and culture, denoting the idea of life force energy. Life force energy is the imperceptible animating property that both embodies and imbues all living things. It reflects both cause and effect. The wind is a perfect metaphor. You can't see it, but you can surely see and feel its material effects. There are many common examples to help us grasp the elusive Eastern concept of energy. For example, we've all been in the presence of someone who's repressing powerful emotions that he or she is attempting to conceal. In spite of this person's failed attempts to repress and conceal, we can't help but feel the energy emanating from those pent-up emotions. This example underscores the great dichotomy of energy, as it is immaterial and imperceptible, yet undeniably powerful. It is the potential of its power that makes this esoteric understanding of energy so compelling.

The power of energy has been studied extensively in the East. Though elusive, the remarkable potentials of energy have been harnessed and channeled in both the martial and healing arts for thousands of years. Acupuncture, acupressure, qigong, Reiki, tai chi, kung fu, karate, and yoga—among many other systems of healing and self-defense—are living testaments to the extraordinary potentials of energy.

Everything is energy, and energy is everywhere. It is always right where it belongs, in its natural place holding the universe together. If we were to pluck even a single particle of energy from the ether in front of our face, the entire universe would collapse. Energy is within us and all around us. It is in infinite supply and always readily available. We have energy within every particle, atom, molecule, chromosome, cell, tissue, and organ of our body. We are all the donors and recipients of a constant flow of life force energy. We receive it from the air we breathe, the food we eat, the love we share, the sun, the moon, and the stars. We are conduits of universal energy that can have too much, just enough, or not enough energy in virtually every given measure of our being. There are times when we might feel that our body has an abundance of energy, even though our spirit feels low. We may begin our day with a depressed spirit but meet up with a good friend later that day who inspires, uplifts, and infuses our psyche. Energy is in a constant state of flux—it is never fixed but always fluid. Its fluidity is clearly observable in our health. One year may be remembered as a period of excellent health with very few episodes of illness, while another reflects a time of frequent doctor visits, nagging symptoms, and absentee days from work. Moreover, the flux that relates to our health energies reveals patterns about our ups and downs. For instance, we may note that our dietary and sleep patterns are healthier during the good years, and not so healthy during the bad years. This overly simplistic example underscores the fact that we have a choice as to whether or not we will cultivate abundant life force energy. The life force energy that brings abundant life and health can be cultivated, generated, intensified, reduced, received, and transmitted. And while our Western minds haven't been formatted to fully appreciate, respect, and implement life force energy as an agent of health and healing, the East provides us with some truly remarkable models for our edification.

A number of years ago, I had the opportunity to observe Chinese doctors in a Beijing hospital perform surgery to remove a brain tumor. Only three physicians were present for the procedure. There was a surgeon, an acupuncturist in charge of anesthesia, and a second acupuncturist to regulate the patient's bleeding. All anesthesia and all hemostatic function were regulated by acupuncture alone. As I looked on, the surgeon actually conversed with the patient throughout the surgery, while the patient's pain and bleeding were completely controlled by needles strategically placed in vital bioenergetic pathways on his body. So, here we see a remarkable example of how the energies associated with pain, bleeding, and vital functions can be regulated and balanced. It was a truly astounding thing to see such energy mastery!

On another occasion, I observed a martial arts qigong master demonstrate a Shaolin self-defense technique, as he effortlessly cast six large attackers to the ground from some thirty feet away. And as they tried to get up, the would-be attackers found themselves frozen to the ground, completely unable to rise. To think, the master was able to do all this with energy. Impressing the mechanistic

Western mind with the sensational potentials of energy only serves as a distraction since, given that mind-set, this form of energy manipulation could only be a trick. But energy isn't merely something we can learn to master. It is rather what we truly are. In fact, it's what everything is—and that's the key point. Energy is about transforming our self-limiting, obsolete material reality, and awakening to energetic reality while opening ourselves up to energy's limitless possibilities.

Nobel Prize–winning physicists have proven that material reality is but a grand illusion. So, too, then, is the notion of limitation that accompanies it. Therefore, it's not merely time we shed our anachronistic material mentality, but also high time we embraced the boundless continuum of possibility that accompanies energetic reality.

The key word once again is "balance." When it comes to the manifestation of energy, there are only three primary manifestations—too much, not enough, and balanced. Both the disharmony of the East and the disease of the West result from either too much or not enough energy.

The primary goal of the WHD is to assess, balance, and preserve energy through its system of energy diagnostics, diet, lifestyle, and mental and emotion management. This can be achieved through energy exercises. Energetically speaking, all aspects of our total being (body, mind, and spirit) are holistically interrelated and interdependent. In order to attain holism and balance, the energies that seek to flow freely within us must be constantly assessed, balanced, and preserved. This is especially true of metabolism and diet.

In the World of Energy, One Size Doesn't Fit All

It's truly remarkable to think that of the seven billion inhabitants of planet earth, no two of them have the same DNA. In spite of this fact, our present culture insists on conducting its affairs as if everyone was the same.

And so it is with our approach to dieting.

Despite the fact that there are three metabolic categories and an infinite array of unique chemistries and personalities, massive numbers of us continue to eat the same diets. We insist on subscribing to this oversimplistic, one-size-fits-all approach to living, but it simply doesn't work, and it never will. In fact, it's one of the major reasons why diets don't work. The only way a dietary program can provide lasting results is if it embraces the philosophy of bio-individuality. Even better by far would be a dietary program that embraces an energy-based individuality. For, far beyond our biological singularity at our unseen core, we are made up of energies that are even more profoundly unique. The differentness of our deeper thoughts, emotions, wishes, hopes, and dreams reveals joined code with separate universes unto themselves.

Energy Codes

I've lived and practiced in New England for many years, and the temperature here ranges seasonally from approximately minus twenty degrees to over one hundred degrees Fahrenheit. Whether we're talking about the temperature variances here in New England, NBA basketball scores, or the amount of calories in different servings of food, there is always a vast but finite number of comparative variables in the material world. In the world of energy, it's very different. In the world of energy, there are but five categories of comparative variables, each with infinite possibilities. These five manifestations of energy are:

1. Abundant
2. Excessive
3. Balanced
4. Deficient
5. Insufficient

Everything in the universe—which includes you and me—has a general energy tendency, or code, that correlates with one of these five manifestations. That is to say, you and I are generally filled with either abundant energy, excessive energy, balanced energy, deficient energy, or insufficient energy. Regarding the aspect of infinite possibilities, the same comparative variables may be assigned to each and every aspect of our lives. For example, someone could have a general constitutional code that is deficient in energy, but when it comes to going to sleep at night, she could be filled with such an excess of energy that she can't sleep. Some people have a strong, energized mind but a deficient, hypersensitive stomach. For our purposes in this book, we will be focusing strictly on your metabolic energy code. This can be initiated by first converting the results of your metabolic questionnaire in chapter 3 into one of the five manifestations of energy. Did you score fast, balanced, or slow? Extremely fast metabolic types should be coded "excessive." Moderately fast metabolic types should be coded "abundant." Balanced metabolic types should be coded "balanced." Moderately slow metabolic types should be coded "deficient." And extremely slow metabolic types should be coded "insufficient."

This little mental exercise is designed to change your programming from material to energetic. These references enable you to begin thinking of yourself, your calorie-burning thyroid gland, and your foods as more than just cellular entities. They provide you with the references and guidelines with which to engage your WHD body, mind, and spirit energy applications.

Energy Dieting

The WHD represents a revolutionary concept that begins with the personal transformation of the dieter. The most important aspect of this personal transformation begins with a redefining of the person's understanding of life—especially self—and food. Up until now, both you and the foods you eat have likely been thought of in the purely material perspective. From this point forward, the WHD requires that you think of yourself and the foods you eat as pure energy. You and I have been conditioned to believe in a material-based reality, even though quantum mechanics has demonstrated that everything appearing to us as matter—including ourselves and the foods we eat—is in fact composed of 99.999 percent energy and only 0.001 percent matter. In fact, everything you see before you is made up of unseen energy particles that mass together, giving the appearance of solid matter. It's not unlike how the freezing of fluid water makes it into solid ice cubes. Both we and the foods we eat are made up of fluid energy that forms solid matter.

There are distinct advantages associated with this transformational shift in perception. The biggest advantage comes from the concept of energetic individuality. By this, I mean every dieter is unique and every food is unique. In the material world all dieters are the same and, once categorized, all foods are also very similar. A dieter is a dieter and a blueberry is a blueberry. In the world of energy, every dieter is unique, and every blueberry is unique—this concept flies in the face of the present one-size-fits-all philosophy. Another decided advantage is that when people follow the guidance of an energy-based dietary system, their ongoing life changes can be more accurately kept up with.

Energy is in a constant state of flux. A dieter who has an efficient calorie-burning metabolism on Monday may encounter an emotionally stressful confrontation on Monday night, which impairs his or her metabolism on Tuesday. Stressful occasions, nightmares, mental anticipation, and joyous excitation are all representative of states that continually weave their way in and out of our lives. These states represent fluctuating shifts in our energies, capable of altering the body's calorie-burning potential. Once mastered, the WHD system enables individuals to bioenergetically pinpoint their most metabolically efficient foods. Equally important, it enables them to keep up with their day-to-day changes with remarkable accuracy.

Optimizing Calorie-Burning Efficiency with Energy

By better understanding energy and the concept of holistic balance, we can better support our metabolism. For our purposes in this book, it's important to note that the energy of our thyroid gland determines the efficiency with which we burn calories. In other words, the more balanced the energy of our thyroid gland, the more efficiently we are likely to metabolize food, burn calories, and stabilize our weight. This all-important balance can be achieved by performing simple energy exercises. With the help of these exercises, anyone can easily channel energy to balance and optimize their metabolic thyroid efficiency. I realize that most of you have likely never heard this before, and it may sound too good to be true. However, all that's necessary is your open mind, your willingness to change, and just a little bit of know-how.

A number of things can deplete the thyroid gland of its energy. Trauma, stress, lack of sleep, improper diet, tobacco, overconsumption of alcoholic beverages, and chronic negative thinking are all capable of depleting a thyroid gland and sending it way out of balance. Remember, energy enters the body and energy is released from the body. When it enters the body, it charges it. When it is released from the body, it depletes it. It's important that we learn to monitor our calorie-burning thyroid energy so that we can recharge it whenever necessary.

Monitoring is quite simple. It begins with simply tuning. I'd like to ask you right now to just take a moment to scan your body's energy field with your mind. Chances are excellent that you can easily tap into the energy state of your thyroid gland by simply tuning in to the field of your vitality. Let's give it a try.

Focus your mind's attention on the energy within your internal body. As you're reading these words I'll ask you to focus your awareness on the zone between your throat and your heart. Do you feel this region between your throat and heart is energetically out of balance, and if so, how? Try to tune in to whether this zone feels hyperenergized, balanced, or exhausted. You might consider repeating the subtle exercise at different times of the day. Remember, energy is always in a state of flux. Nonetheless, the more you practice this monitoring process, the more it will enable you to zero in on your energy code.

The Power of Thought-Field Energy

So, if everything is energy, then all energy must exist within a certain domain. The area occupied by any given concentration of energy is called a field. For example, we've all seen photographs of lightning strikes, revealing ambient energy charges encircling jagged bolts of lightning. The human electromagnetic field generally produces an aura that extends from the body to a distance of between one and thirty-six inches. Everything is energy, and all energy manifests within a concentrated field. Every particle produces an energy field. Every atom produces an energy field. Every molecule produces an energy field. Every strand of DNA produces an energy field. Every cell produces an energy field. Every vital tissue produces an energy field. Every gland and organ produce an energy field. Therefore, your thyroid gland produces an active energy field that expands and contracts depending on trauma, stress, diet, and sleep, among other factors. As previously stated, energy represents both cause and effect. Not only are we made up of energy, but we are also capable of altering energy. Moreover, we are capable of being a conduit, channeling energy for the purpose of balancing. So if your thyroid energy is deficient, you may channel energy into it for the purpose of strengthening and balancing. If your thyroid is overactive, you may decrease its excessive energy in order to bring it into a state of better balance.

This is actually quite simple. It's all about projecting a strong channel of energy via intention. We must remember that thoughts are things and that energy and matter are interconvertible. We merely have to overcome the confusing limitations imposed by our material indoctrination. By combining strong mental intention with determined willpower, we are amassing powerful energy that must ultimately be converted into matter. Perhaps Einstein summarized it best by simply stating, "Energy creates matter." Simply focus your thoughts on the area at the base of your neck, just underneath your Adam's apple. This is the area occupied by your thyroid gland. Then visualize yourself transmitting a healing stream of balanced energy from the brow area between your eyes directly to your thyroid gland, for no more than two to three minutes. For anyone who is overweight or obese or who has been diagnosed with thyroid disease, this exercise should be practiced daily.

Energetically Thinking Yourself Thin

The hypothesis that human consciousness has the potential to directly affect matter in the form of metabolism change and weight loss represents a considerable stretch for most material minds, but cutting-edge quantum physics provides more than one detailed explanation.

The theory of orchestrated objective reduction, recently advanced by mathematical physicist Sir Roger Penrose and anesthesiologist Stuart Hameroff, asserts that the energy of human consciousness vibrates materially within the microtubules of brain neurons.[2] This recent groundbreaking research, published in *Physics of Life Reviews*, identifies the genesis where the ether of thought first metamorphoses into the biological, and opens the door to a fuller understanding of how thought energy alters matter.

Human thought produces anharmonic vibrations within brain-neuron microtubules, which are then transferred between synapses—but the vibrational frequency they emit generates much more than a mere local influence. Our thoughts produce frequencies that are transmitted into the infinite. Every thought we think changes the universe, particle by particle. According to the laws of superposition, our observation of reality has a direct effect on reality. We must keep two important points in mind here—first, that everything is energy; and second, that thoughts are things. In fact, thoughts are energetic things that make material things happen.

"Max Planck, Hubbard, Einstein, and Stephen Hawking all seem to agree that the universe/god is actually a set of laws and principles that we can count on to create our world," writes author Peter Baksa. "Stephen Hawking and Richard Feynman both speak in terms of M-theory and string theory to further postulate how thoughts become matter. Our minds are essentially idea machines, that refine our thoughts into electrical impulses, which communicate with the same source energy that creates everything from nothing."[3] Therefore, by the mere nature of our consciousness, we are creators. So how, then, might we create changes in our physical metabolism with our conscious thoughts? Over the years, I've instructed thousands of patients in the art of thinking themselves thin. It's always proved helpful and it's really quite simple.

Both our thyroid gland and our thoughts are made up of energy. Our thoughts are made up of energy that possesses the power to create material change. It's all about setting a strong intention to have an effect. Remember, there are three major options for energy. Energy is either deficient, balanced, or excessive. If our thyroid gland is underactive, and we've always struggled to lose weight, it means that our thyroid is energy deficient. If our thyroid energy is deficient, we might consider setting a strong thought intention designed to boost our thyroid gland, and thus our calorie-burning potential. This isn't rocket science. I advise patients to take four minutes in the morning and four minutes in the afternoon to sit in a quiet, undisturbed environment, with eyes closed, while engaging in positive willful thoughts determined to stimulate their thyroid gland, located at the front base of the neck. Simply send it some determined, energy-charged thoughts twice daily for four minutes each time, and make things happen meta-bolically.

The Power of Imagination Energy

In the words of Albert Einstein, "Imagination is more important than knowledge. Knowledge is limited. Imagination encircles the world."

"Einstein's aphorism reflects a recurrent theme in human thought," writes Prashjay. "The ancient dichotomy between what we know and what we dream is found, in some form, in every field of human intellectual endeavor."[4]

He taught us that energy and matter are two manifestations of the same thing. We might do well to think of energy as activated matter, and matter as energy waiting to be activated. Everything is energy, even us, every scintilla of us. Our body, mind, and spirit are made up of both activated energy and energy waiting to be activated. Our ability to activate our matter into energy is limited only by our belief. Our perception about our capacity to have an energetic effect on ourselves, each other, the world, and the universe is grossly underestimated. Our programming has led us to believe the only real effects we're capable of producing are those tangible, material effects that are aligned with our five senses. We know we can effect material change with the power of our hands, but what about the power of our imagination? After all, imagination represents the creative ability to form a picture of something in our mind that eludes the senses. Imagination is often a form of highly inspired thought, or thought in spirit.

Like all things, conscious thought is composed of energy. So every time we imagine, we create. Thoughts are things. Our mechanistically programmed minds tend to have a hard time associating the imperceptible nature of thought as something tangible. However, we must keep in mind that thought has crystalline, quartzlike properties that generate electromagnetic frequencies, capable of altering matter.

Ongoing neuroplasticity research continues to discover that rehearsed imagination is a primary vehicle for the brain's neurogenesis. In other words, the more frequently we imagine an event, the more our brain redesigns and adapts itself to support its manifestation. Translation: imagine it often enough, and you likely create it. Neuroplasticity studies have shown that whenever we focus on an intention, we activate neural pathways in the brain in a way that can actually increase the outcome probability.

A 2004 study performed by the Cleveland Clinic discovered that subjects could increase their finger strength 53 percent through physical exercise over a twelve-week period. Remarkably, a second group in the study showed a 35 percent strength increase through mental visualization alone.[5] According to a 2007 study performed at Bishop's University in Quebec, athletes who practiced hip flexor exercises increased muscle strength 28 percent. Astoundingly, a second group was able to increase the same hip flexor strength 24 percent by simply imagining that they were practicing the same hip flexor exercises.[6]

A 2007 Harvard study led by neurologist Alvaro Pascual-Leone gave a group of musically skilled subjects instructions to practice a specific piece for five days, two hours a day, for a total of ten hours. Their brains were scanned before and after each practice session. As expected, the skilled subjects revealed active neural stimulation in a part of the brain called the anterior cingulate cortex. Another group, made up of randomly selected, musically unskilled subjects, was given almost the same exact assignment. The only difference between the two groups was that the unskilled musicians never actually physically played the piano—instead, they engaged in mental rehearsal only. They, too, were brain scanned before and after each rehearsal session. Pascual-Leone and his associates were amazed to discover that the results of the brain scans consistently revealed exactly the same active neural brain stimulation with the mental rehearsal group as with the physical performance group.[7] Because of this, and other similar studies, researchers have come to learn that the anterior cingulate cortex responds to imagination exactly as it responds to fact. Simply put, it believes what it sees. Moreover, by simply visualizing an event, the anterior cingulate cortex cues the rest of the body to physiologically respond to the imagined visualization as if it were real.

Might this phenomenon prove useful to dieters?

In 2010, Carey Morewedge, then an assistant professor of social and decision sciences at Carnegie Mellon University, led three hundred volunteers in an interesting imagination study that showed that by imagining eating a food, we tend to reduce our actual consumption of that food. In fact, Morewedge and his associates noted a reduction of 50 percent in the amount of food consumed by participants who imagined eating that food before actually being given it.[8]

The neurological processes of our brain's anterior cingulate cortex determine what is called "habituation." Habituation is described as our mechanistic approach to determining how much one is in fact overconsuming beyond the satiety point. So, by simply imagining (visualizing) that you are overconsuming food, your brain will kick into habituation mode, convincing your body that it's had enough.

The WHD encourages dieters to devote a minimum of ten minutes per day to a visualization exercise in which they envision themselves overconsuming a favorite food. When I first introduce this idea to many of my patients, they often express great apprehension, thinking that it will increase their consumption. I encourage them not to be afraid, and I remind them that this exercise has proven extremely helpful to many thousands of WHD dieters over the past three decades.

CHAPTER 6

OUR ENERGY GUIDANCE SYSTEM (EGS)

Intuitive Intelligence

Are you in touch with your extrasensory perception (ESP)? According to a recent Gallup Poll, 41 percent of Americans believe in ESP, yet most doubt that they possess any intuitive skills. But science now tells us that it's more likely a matter of your not using those skills than not having them. In fact, not only do you possess intuitive smarts, you've been developing them for a long time.

Researchers from the University of Missouri Developmental Cognition Lab have proven that the human brain is indeed intuitively adroit. Moreover, ongoing studies reveal that we're all precognitively wired at around the age of two months. The researchers point out that infant precognition is most likely developed before the age of two months, but because testing can't be effectively administered on infants until that time, it can't be confirmed. Therefore, the fact of the matter is that science has definitively confirmed that we human beings are fully equipped for intuitive function shortly after our birth, and quite possibly even earlier. Once again, it's less about not having it and more about not using it. Then again, you're not inclined to use something you don't know you have.

Ours is a mechanistic cultural experiment. Our reality baselines are tightly affixed to systems and concepts born of structure and control. We've been programmed to align everything we think and do with the ordered cultural framework that's been set in place. This greater framework serves as a guideline for what we're to believe is possible. Our Western minds weren't fashioned to comprehend extrasensory phenomena.

Phenomena may simply be defined as "extra-ordinary" experiences. When you consider the infinite realm of both natural and quantum phenomena in the world, solar system, universe, multiverse, and cosmos, there's very little that's "ordinary." Once again, rooted within our instinct to survive is a "shrink things down to my size" mentality. It's this "survival" mind-set that says, "If I can't slow things down to my level of comprehension, I'll just put them aside because they're too laborious."

Intuition represents the extra-ordinary. We might simply refer to it, then, as a form of phenomenon—a phenomenon that we can't shrink down to our size. Because it won't chunk down, we'll just chalk it up as being unreal. It simply doesn't fit our mechanistic cultural model. Nonetheless, it's "out there"—or should I say "in there"—and it refuses to leave us alone.

I just met with a woman who shared an interesting story. She said that she was recently driving through a two-lane one-way tunnel in the greater Boston area marked with a solid double line. She was cruising along at a pretty good speed, hovering in the left lane, when out of the blue something told her to quickly pull over into the right lane. In spite of the fact that the solid lines indicated that it was illegal to switch lanes, she suddenly moved into the right lane, and at the very instant she did, a two-ton pickup truck that was going the wrong way inside the tunnel appeared and rumbled right by her in the travel lane that she'd occupied milliseconds earlier. Whatever it was that told her to pull over likely prevented a head-on collision.

During the early twentieth century, C. G. Jung, a Swiss psychiatrist and the founder of the school of analytical psychology, proposed that human beings have four primary pathways for processing information: thinking, feeling, sensing, and intuiting. This pioneering vision of Jung's has at last blossomed into a whole new world of neuroscientific brain mapping.

Today, brain mapping reveals the extraordinary diversity and infinite capacity of the human brain to process information. The latest research in this area has discovered that our brain knows the decisions we're going to make a full six seconds before we make them. What's more, it's confirmed that this precognitive process is actually a natural part of our brain's biology. Intuition engages both the mind and the body.

"Scientists have discovered that humans appear to have two, very different 'operating systems,'" writes researcher Kelly Turner. "System 1 is our quick, instinctual, and often subconscious way of operating—it is controlled by our right brain and by other parts of our brain that have been around since prehistoric times, known as the 'limbic' and 'reptilian' parts of our brain. System 2 is our slower, more analytical, and conscious way of operating—it is controlled by our left brain and by newer parts of our brain that have only developed since prehistoric times (also known as the 'neocortex'). Researchers have found that intuition is part of System 1, which is why it comes on so rapidly and often does not make rational sense to us. In other words, intuitive decisions are not something that we have thought out carefully with reason, but rather choices that have arisen quickly out of instinct."[1] Intuitive human instinct is now the subject of a great many scientific studies being performed all around the world.

In one study, conducted at the Birth and Women's Health Center in Tucson, Arizona, one hundred pregnant women were asked by a research team to predict whether they would give birth to a boy or girl. Those women planning to exercise intuition to try to determine the gender of their child made the right choice over 70 percent of the time. One of the study's authors, Victor Shamas, explained that pregnant mothers also often use their intuitive ability to tap into other aspects of their baby's identity as well. Shamas goes on to explain that pregnant mothers frequently record premonition-like dreams that accurately predict what kinds of people their children will turn out to be—including specifics like their particular preferences, temperament, and even future careers. Furthermore, he points out that 75 percent of college students he surveyed contended that their mothers were able to read their thoughts and feelings like no one else, while 80 percent said that their mothers were more intuitive than their fathers.[2]

Intuition represents a delicate balance between not only the brain and the mind, but the heart as well.

According to recent findings of a new prestimulus response study performed at the HeartMath Institute, heart rate variability represents a reliable means of measuring intuitive intelligence.

Subjects participated in a gambling experiment and were encouraged to win as much as possible over the full course of twenty-six trials. "For each trial, electrodes were attached to the pads of participants' index and second fingers of their nondominant hands so skin conductance levels could be measured, and electrocardiographic information was recorded from electrodes placed on the chest so heart-rate variability/HRV (the beat-to-beat changes in heart rate) could be recorded. They chose bet amounts and then selected either *red* or *black* for each impending spin of the roulette wheel on a computer screen. The resulting color for each spin was compared to participants' color choices.

According to Rollin McCraty, director of the HMI Research Center, "The heart-rhythm measures (HRV) were especially successful in detecting pre-stimulus responses in the pre-bet and post-bet segments. . . . [T]he difference in the win/loss response was evident some 12–14 seconds before the result *red* or *black* was made known to the participant.

"We also found that a greater heart-rate deceleration was predictive of losing trials in the pre-bet segment, and the divergence in the win/loss curve begins almost immediately after starting the trials, which on average occurs around 18 seconds prior to knowing the future outcome."[3]

Those of us who are more philosophically mechanistic by nature are not inclined to believe in the existence of a sixth sense. Paradoxically, if we don't believe, it can't possibly exist. Our sixth sense is a little bit like a muscle. If you don't use it, you lose it.

When I first began my work more than thirty years ago, I didn't subcribe to the belief in any such thing as innate, intuitive intelligence. However, I gradually started to experiment with the idea and ultimately incorporated elements of what I was finding into my work. As time went on, my dabbling became more routine and my results more consistent. I would've never believed that I would one day develop a comprehensive healing system based on innate, intuitive intelligence. Since then, I've had the pleasure of teaching my Whole Health system to thousands of allied health care specialists, including neurosurgeons, physicians, nurse practitioners, osteopaths, chiropractors, and acupuncturists. The allied professionals, office associates, and interns that I've trained have consistently been able to obtain the same effective results by learning to tap into innate, intuitive intelligence.

Our Energy Guidance System (EGS)

The WHD distinguishes itself from every other diet by teaching the dieter how to identify the most efficient calorie-burning foods for his or her body—and his or her body alone. Clearly not just another one-size-fits-all diet program, the WHD presents dieters with three important concepts that will enable them to calibrate and customize their diet for maximum efficiency. The first of these is the concept of an energy guidance system (EGS). The term "energy guidance system" refers to our innate, intuitive intelligence. The concept of innate intelligence was first advanced by Daniel David Palmer, father of modern chiropractic medicine. He described it as the force responsible for the organizing, maintaining, and healing of the human body. Some experts now theorize that innate intelligence first appears during human fertilization, ultimately accounting for the precise differentiation of embryonic stem cells into two distinct cell lines. This innate force of intelligence that directs our genetic differentiation is anything but random. With near perfect consistency, heart cells somehow know to become part of the heart, brain cells somehow know to become part of the brain, and fingers somehow know not to become toes.

The WHD recognizes that there is an innate intelligence that acts as a guiding force, common to all nature, that's readily observable. For example, when you water your plants, you may notice that they know to turn their least exposed leaves directly into the highest saturation of sunlight. Similarly, the trees, shrubs, and flowering plants in your yard always seem to know exactly how to best position themselves for the highest amount of direct sunlight. Innate intelligence provides an energy guidance system for the entire animal kingdom as well. Homing pigeons are known to find their way home over distances of nearly 1,200 miles, while maintaining speeds of over fifty miles per hour. Researchers have found this to be true time and time again, even when the pigeons are transported to distant places they've never visited before. Experts theorize that the pigeon's innate navigation system comprises olfactory sensors, light-mediated mechanisms in the brain, and iron particles in the beak, believed to keep it magnetically aligned with true north.

The WHD teaches that since we are energy beings with the capacity for extrasensory awareness, we are all equipped with a built-in energy guidance system. In fact, our EGS is present and active every moment of our lives—we're just not always aware of it. At the biological level, our EGS governs our breathing and heart rate. Also, it might be simply thought of as an instinctual hunch. For example, whenever we attempt to cross a busy street in the middle of a city block, we'll wait until we get a strong sense as to when it is safest to make a run for it. We may have a hunch that a friend or loved one is in need of our attention in a special way, only to find that the person contacts us later that same day. Our energy guidance system is continually getting hunches, which typically go unnoticed.

Within our bodies there's a constant flow of communication being exchanged between cells. Half of this communication is reflective of logic, and half is reflective of intuition. Our innate cell-to-cell communication system originates in our heart—more specifically, a bundle of afferent nerves within our heart called the intrinsic cardiac ganglia. This has been identified by scientists as an extrasensory perception and communication center within the heart. It's also often referred to as the "little brain" in the heart, as it not only has the ability to think and communicate, but has actually been identified as the originator of much of our innate thinking. You see, for many years scientists believed that all origination of thought took place exclusively in the big brain, but thanks in large part to the remarkable research of Dr. J. Andrew Armour of the HeartMath Institute in Boulder Creek, California, founded in 1991, we now know otherwise. Armour discovered that the little brain within the heart actually initiates the majority of our thought and cell-to-cell communication, as it signals the big brain to relay information to the rest of the body. This is especially true when it comes to our innate, intuitive awareness. The intrinsic cardiac ganglia bundle is the signaling center of our energy guidance system, the origin of all our hunches and extrasensory perceptions. One might say that this is the place where "we simply know in our hearts what's true."

So the little brain within the heart is the home base of your innate energy guidance system. This extrasensory information center is always turned on; it never shuts off. Furthermore, it's easy to tap into because it's a biofeedback loop that's wired from the heart to the brain and on through to the nerves and muscles. So when it comes to being able to tap into your own intuitive information with consistent reliability, your nerves and muscles are the perfect medium. As we shall see shortly, muscle testing the WHD way enables practitioners to easily and accurately tap into their own energy guidance system for the purposes of really homing in on the customizing and personalizing of their diet plan. The WHD Electromagnetic Muscle Testing system allows dieters to access information from their energy guidance system in a way that will help them to clearly identify the optimal foods capable of maximizing their metabolism.

Electromagnetic Feedback

The word "feedback" is common to our lexicon. It is generally translated as an answer, an observation, or a reaction. Regarding the world of health care, diagnosis is the most important form of feedback, as it helps us to arrive at the solution by first determining how the problem came about.

Mathematician Norbert Wiener, winner of the National Medal of Science, is perhaps best noted for his cybernetics theory, which proposed that living systems may be controlled by monitoring their results. In 1969, participants at a landmark conference in Santa Monica, California, were the first to come up with the term "biofeedback," which they say was inspired by the work of Norbert Wiener. Today, biofeedback is playing a significant role in health care. "Biofeedback is a technique you can use to learn to control your body's functions, such as your heart rate," explains staff at the Mayo Clinic. "With biofeedback, you're connected to electrical sensors that help you receive information (feedback) about your body (bio). This feedback helps you focus on making subtle changes in your body, such as relaxing certain muscles, to achieve the results you want, such as reducing pain. In essence, biofeedback gives you the power to use your thoughts to control your body, often to help with a health condition or physical performance."[4]

There are two approaches to practicing medicine: intervention and prevention. Without biofeedback, there can be no preventive medicine. Any effective practice of preventive medicine demands as much vital information about a subject's health tendencies as can be obtained. The more that can be learned about a patient's constitutional deficiencies and health tendencies, the more likely that preventive strategies may be successfully invoked to prevent probabilities from becoming outcomes. Therefore, central to effective prevention is the idea of setting up a feedback loop between the mind and the body. This is precisely what muscle testing is all about, but instead of providing biofeedback, it provides electromagnetic feedback. Where biofeedback is matter based, electromagnetic feedback is energy based. Also, biofeedback monitoring typically requires state-of-the-art biomedical equipment capable of measuring brain waves, blood pressure, dermal response, concentration, memory, and immunity to stress. Electromagnetic feedback requires only a subject, a partner, and a little basic training.

Electromagnetic feedback is an excellent way for one to glean information about the status of one's metabolism, thyroid function, and calorie-burning potential. Electromagnetic Muscle Testing (EMT) is a well-designed system for determining the energetic strengths and weaknesses of our calorie-burning machinery. It is also an excellent means for discovering which specific food energies most strengthen and weaken an individual's metabolic energy (Acutrition). In addition, EMT represents a fluid feedback system capable of keeping up with the constant changes that our bodies experience.

Electromagnetic Muscle Testing (EMT)

Electromagnetic Muscle Testing is a reliable means by which we can tap into our EGS, in order to obtain vital feedback from the source of our innate wisdom. In the material world, the primary source of all guidance and information is the "other," not the innate "self." We've learned well not to trust the instinctual wisdom of self. Instead, we've been taught to seek out the calculated logic of the world. This is especially true in the areas of health care and weight loss. But we know much more than we think. Once we tap into our wellspring of instinctual wisdom with the help of muscle testing, an entire universe of information will open up to us. I shall not soon forget the first time I had the good fortune to work with muscle testing. Like most people, I was completely taken aback by my nervous system's remarkable responsiveness, as well as my neuromuscular accuracy. I remember thinking, "Why should I be so surprised at my own receptiveness and precision?" After all, our nervous system is made up of neuroelectrical pathways that flow through our muscles. Along with my astonishment, I remember feeling resentful that I had been so systematically denied my own innate knowledge for so many years. When efficiently administered, muscle testing is a remarkable tool that empowers us with the ability to clearly and consistently tune in to our own innate answers. Thus, when it comes to the question of who has the perfect design for your optimal personalized diet plan, the answer is—you do! You just may not know it yet, because you, too, have been systematically indoctrinated to deny your own inner knowledge.

The Electromagnetic Muscle Testing system that's part of the Whole Health healing system is the cornerstone of the WHD. It's what separates it from any other diet plan, as it equips dieters with the ability to individualize and update their diet plan for maximum efficiency.

For more comprehensive instructions and analysis of EMT, refer to my previous book *Whole Health: A Holistic Approach to Healing for the 21st Century*.

For our purposes in this book, we will concentrate on the following five EMT applications: positioning, pass/fail testing, tuning, pulse testing, and focus/reliability testing. These five represent the basic EMT techniques that form the bases of the tests that follow.

1. EMT POSITIONING. EMT requires two people: the "practitioner," or tester, and the "subject." Practitioner and subject begin by standing face-to-face, approximately arm's length apart from each other. Both partners must have their feet spread about shoulder-width apart for stability. The practitioner will use his or her dominant hand in the test. The subject raises his or her opposite arm (the left, if the practitioner is right-handed) out to the side, to slightly higher than shoulder height. Make sure to extend the arm straight out with no bend in the elbow. The subject should then clench the fist and tighten up the arm so as to gently resist as the practitioner attempts to push down on the subject's extended wrist. Both partners must see to it that their posture remains erect.

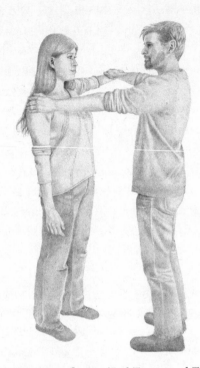

EMT Positioning for Pass/Fail Testing and Tuning

2. EMT PASS/FAIL TESTING. Now you're ready to conduct your first pass/fail test. Begin by having the practitioner hold a small sugar packet directly on the chest of the subject, approximately in front of the heart. Once the sugar

packet is in place, the practitioner should give a light and sturdy push on the subject's wrist. This baseline pass/fail test should consistently make the subject's arm go down easily. This result is called a "failure." Now, take three to five minutes to get comfortable with your positioning.

3. EMT TUNING. Once you both have taken the time to get comfortable with positioning, posture, and strength differential, it's time for tuning. Your aim here is to make sure that you're both on the same page and in sync with each other for an efficient pass/fail testing experience. Once again, practitioner and subject must stand before each other in the proper EMT positioning. Practitioner: begin by calling out a negative word, like "sickness," while at the same time performing a pass/fail muscle test on the subject. Merely hearing the negative word will cause the subject's energy field and neuromuscular strength to be diminished, generally producing a failed muscle test. Remember, words alone generate energy that affects our strength. Negative words produce negative energy, and positive words produce positive energy. Don't be afraid to choose other negative words, like "misery," "hopelessness," or "disease," and to administer the test more than once in order to establish a clear-cut failed muscle response.

Next, repeat the exact same procedure, but now you should call out a positive word, like "happiness." Once again, don't hesitate to run this test more than once while calling out other positive words, such as "healthy," "vibrant," or "blissful." The key here is to establish a definitively strong muscle test response (a "passing" result) that stands in clear contrast to the subject's previous failed response. Tuning is extremely important for establishing an accurate baseline between practitioner and subject. Once you've mastered EMT pass/fail testing, it's time for you to go on to pulse testing.

4. EMT PULSE TESTING. This technique allows practitioner and subject to pinpoint the exact relative plus-or-minus score of their pass/fail test results. In other words, where pass/fail testing allows you only to establish a pass or fail result, pulse testing enables you to calibrate the exact degree of your plus or minus result. For example, if a subject's muscle strength passed after being pulse tested for a given positive word, you can then measure the exact degree of the positive reaction along a relative range of plus 1 to plus 10. A pulse test score of plus 10 would indicate a stronger positive reaction than a pulse test score of plus 1.

The same pulse testing method can be applied to a negative response as well, using the range minus 1 to minus 10, with minus 10 being a stronger negative reaction. It's also important to note here that practitioner and subject have the option of using unlimited numbers, instead of restricting the maximum value to 10. This energy testing modality is nothing more than a neuromuscular biofeedback vehicle that allows us to tap into our stream of innate consciousness. We can set the intention as we so choose. I highly recommend pulse testing in unlimited numbers from time to time.

Here's how it works. Remember, pulse testing is a follow-up to pass/fail testing. Therefore, prior to engaging in pulse testing, let's assume that the subject has just failed a pass/fail test upon hearing the word "sickness." The

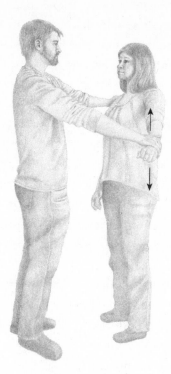

EMT Pulse Testing

practitioner should then state aloud the intention to pulse test the subject for exactly how negatively the word "sickness" affects the subject's energy, on a scale between minus 1 and minus 10. The practitioner should then call out the word "sickness" once again, but this time, instead of pushing straight down on the subject's arm once, as in the pass/fail test, the practitioner will gently pulse, or push down repeatedly on the subject's wrist, while simultaneously counting aloud from minus 1 to minus 10.

If the subject's arm strength weakens and fails at a pulse count between minus 5 and minus 10, this should be considered a severe negative energetic reaction. Test scores between minus 1 and minus 5 should therefore be considered less severe.

Practitioner and subject can apply this same pulse testing technique to measure the subject's positive responses, from plus 1 to plus 10, as well.

Pulse testing is the most important feature of the entire WHD plan. As you'll soon discover, EMT pulse testing is the technique that makes the difference, enabling dieters to zero in on the ongoing health status of their thyroid gland, as well as the optimal foods and food supplements to efficiently fuel their calorie-burning metabolism. EMT pulse testing is the secret weapon that allows each dieter to accurately map out his or her individual, personalized diet plan. Moreover, it makes it possible for dieters to keep up with their ever-changing dietary needs at a very subtle level.

5. FOCUS/RELIABILITY TESTING. This is an additional pulse testing protocol designed to ensure focus, concentration, and reliability between practitioner and subject. Once again, the practitioner and subject stand in the basic EMT positioning for pass/fail testing. The practitioner should state the question, "What is our present degree of focus and reliability, from plus 1 to plus 10, with plus 10 representing 100 percent?" The two should then immediately

perform a pulse test, counting from plus 1 to plus 10. If the subject's pulse test score is less than 5, then practitioner and subject should take a moment to gather their wits and rededicate their concentration efforts. A simple deep cleansing breath, a momentary time-out, is typically more than enough to get you both back on track. Next, simply repeat pulse testing. You should notice the numbers elevate. If not, just take a few more moments to re-group, then retest.

Metabolic Testing

One of the main goals of the Whole Health Diet is to provide the readers with some basic energy tools to help them better manage metabolism and support weight loss. Up to this point you've had an Electromagnetic Muscle Testing primer and should now be ready to move on to the Six Metabolic Tests format. This format begins with basic Rudiment Testing, and then goes on to teach you how to energetically test the strength of your thyroid gland, as well as your thyroid response to specific foods. It also teaches you how to construct a personalized meal and supplement plan that's best suited to maximize your weight loss potential.

The Six Metabolic EMT Tests:

1. Rudiment testing
2. Thyroid energy testing

3. Food energy testing (Acutrition)
4. Customized meal plan testing
5. Raw versus cooked food testing
6. Nutritional supplement testing

1. RUDIMENT TESTING

My dear friend Dr. Bernie Siegel shared a story with me that I shall never forget. He said he once delivered an address to thousands of terminally ill people. As he concluded his talk, he made the following announcement: "If anyone would like to live longer and be healthier, report to the meeting room down the hall." To his shock and amazement, only ten women showed up. The moral of the story is that most of us are reluctant to make a commitment.

One of the main reasons that dieting has such a high rate of failure is that, while many may claim to want to lose weight, when it comes right down to it, they're not ready to make the necessary commitment. Therefore, it is important to begin by performing an EMT rudiment testing exercise in order to establish the dieter's commitment level right at the outset.

Rudiment testing is quite simple. As with all EMT procedures, subject and practitioner stand arm's length apart. Next, they tune and test for reliability. Once they're tuned and reliable, the subject must then affirmatively state his or her specific goal out loud: "I want to lose [number] pounds!" Immediately following this statement, the two perform an EMT pass/fail muscle test. If the subject is truly ready to perform all that is required, he or she will pass this test. Assuming that is so, they then do a pulse test in order to determine the relative degree of the subject's determination to succeed. If the pulse test registers between 1 and 5, the subject should take some time to go deep within in order to see if he or she can muster a stronger commitment. This is followed by additional pulse testing. If, on the other hand, the subject is truly not ready, he or she will typically fail the muscle test. This may sound like a harsh, negative exercise, but in fact it helps people to tune in to their innermost consciousness, in a way that allows them to reexamine their honest level of commitment. The rudiment test is a quick, easy way to prevent dieting disaster. Moreover, it enables individuals to truly establish the mental intention necessary to successfully complete the task before they get started.

2. THYROID ENERGY TESTING

The energetic state of your thyroid gland is different today from what it was yesterday. Its subtle properties have been affected by myriad energetic influences within and around you. Diet, stress, sleep, hydration, and social interaction have all influenced the energies of your thyroid gland. Once again, material logic has led you to just assume that the thyroid you have today is the same thyroid you had yesterday. The world of energy tells you that nothing could be further from the truth. This underscores the difference-making uniqueness of the WHD program. The EMT thyroid energy testing procedure enables you to assess the exact degree of energetic strength of your thyroid gland, and the food energy testing procedure that follows it provides you with pinpoint accuracy to determine those specific foods that will best energize your thyroid gland, and thus your metabolism. Moreover, these energies that represent you and your metabolism are fluid, not static.

Metabolic thyroid testing calls for the EMT pass/fail and pulse testing tech-

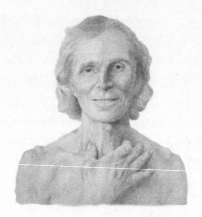

Thyroid energy point

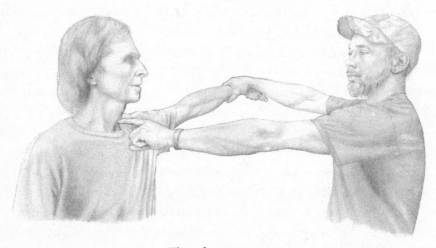

Thyroid energy testing

niques. First, practitioner and subject assume the EMT positioning. Next, practitioner and subject run a few sample pass/fail tests, get themselves properly in tune with each other, and then pulse test for their focus/reliability factor. (If a refresher on how to perform these tests is needed, please refer back to the EMT pass/fail and pulse testing techniques as outlined previously.) Once this preliminary setup work is completed, the partners should be ready to go on to pass/fail and pulse test the strength or weakness of the subject's thyroid gland.

Thyroid energy testing is quite simple. The practitioner and subject perform the EMT pass/fail testing technique followed by the pulse testing technique, *but while performing these two tests, the practitioner places the index finger of his or her nondominant hand on the subject's thyroid gland, directly at the base of the throat.*

This all-important test allows the practitioner and subject to accurately assess the excess, balance, or deficiency of the subject's thyroid gland energy.

3. FOOD ENERGY TESTING (ACUTRITION)

Everything is energy. The thyroid gland represents one form of energy, while food represents another. Any time energies converge, the result is either a positive or a negative reaction. And so it is metabolically. You may not have been aware of it up to this point, but every food you have ever eaten has had a unique energetic effect on your thyroid metabolism. Up until now, you've been programmed to believe that food affects metabolism based solely on material properties. For example, you've been taught that fatty foods and high-starch carbohydrates slow down metabolism, solely because of their molecular density. In contrast, you've been told that lean proteins, low-starch vegetables, and low-sugar fruits stimulate metabolism solely because they're less dense and more activating. So it is with the bias of material logic. But in the world of energy there's a whole other thought process. In theory, each separate blueberry in the container has a unique and different set of energetic properties. Energy is DNA, in the sense that it is sui generis. Energy is also in an ongoing state of flux—it is forever shifting and changing.

EMT food energy testing (Acutrition) is a simple procedure. "Acutrition" is a term that I first coined back in the 1980s. It refers to the "pinpoint, acupuncture accuracy" of the Whole Health nutrition program. It was then that I first began experimenting with the idea of designing energy-based, customized nutrition plans. Even then, I found the concept of one-size-fits-all nutrition so disturbing that I was inspired to develop a system that enabled people to effectively test their energy with the energy of foods, so that they might personalize their approach to dieting. In addition, Acutrition was further designed to help people test the energy of their specific glands or organs for strengths and weaknesses, as well as for their positive and negative reactions to foods, so as to help them zero in on their optimal metabolic nutrition options.

Acutrition was inspired by the concept of energetic individuality and constitutional codes. We are all as unique as snowflakes, yet we continue to put up with the cattle-prodding approach espoused by nutritionists and medical professionals. Most of our ancestral systems of medicine were designed with human constitutional coding in mind. These systems, and the people who developed them, respected the constitutional differences that exist between one person and another. The world and universe were viewed as cosmologies of uniqueness and distinction, where no two people were alike. Subsequently, the food and medicine protocols were uniquely designed to suit each individual's code.

Today, it doesn't seem to occur to us that DNA isn't the only manifestation of our uniqueness. In fact, every particle of energy, atom, and molecule that we're composed of is a reflection of our unique, irreproducible code. The same can be said for all living things, including foods. Consider the fact that there are over one hundred dietary theories today, yet only one of them, the WHD, is energetically designed to match your personal constitutional code.

Thanks to the remarkable EMT system, Acutrition is the key that unlocks the door to your code. By tuning you in to the dynamics of your code at the subtlest energetic level, and by employing the highest elements of your mind-body field of awareness, Acutrition, in combination with EMT, maximizes your ability to attain metabolic balance. When one lives in the state of maximum balance, body weight seeks its natural balance.

The EMT food energy test we'll be performing is referred to as thyroid food exposure testing. It tests the thyroid gland's response to foods. The thyroid food exposure test will enable you to pinpoint all of those foods that support and sabotage your metabolism. You'll be amazed to find that many "healthy" foods, recommended on most diet plans, actually fail EMT testing. This will awaken you to the fact that pinpointed, individualized testing is the only way to truly determine the most ideal, personalized metabolic food plan for your weight loss and optimal health.

Before getting started with EMT food energy testing, practitioner and subject will need to design a Whole Health food classification chart, like the one shown on the next page.

Next, the two can begin by sequencing through EMT positioning and pass/fail testing, followed by pulse testing and tuning.

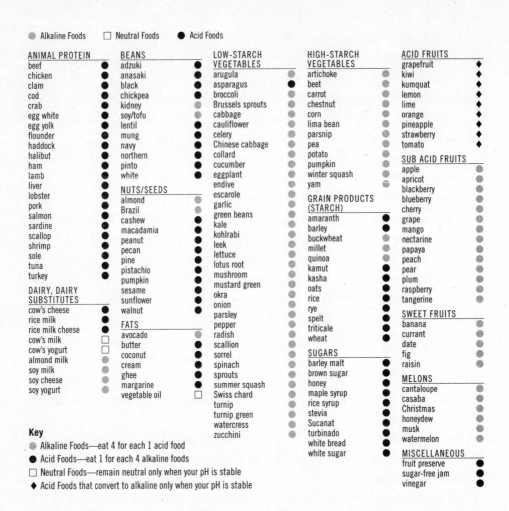

● Alkaline Foods   □ Neutral Foods   ● Acid Foods

ANIMAL PROTEIN
beef ●
chicken ●
clam ●
cod ●
crab ●
egg white ●
egg yolk ●
flounder ●
haddock ●
halibut ●
ham ●
lamb ●
liver ●
lobster ●
pork ●
salmon ●
sardine ●
scallop ●
shrimp ●
sole ●
tuna ●
turkey ●

DAIRY, DAIRY SUBSTITUTES
cow's cheese ●
rice milk ●
rice milk cheese ●
cow's milk □
cow's yogurt □
almond milk ●
soy milk ●
soy cheese ●
soy yogurt ●

BEANS
adzuki ●
anasaki ●
black ●
chickpea ●
kidney ●
soy/tofu ●
lentil ●
mung ●
navy ●
northern ●
pinto ●
white ●

NUTS/SEEDS
almond ●
Brazil ●
cashew ●
macadamia ●
peanut ●
pecan ●
pine ●
pistachio ●
pumpkin ●
sesame ●
sunflower ●
walnut ●

FATS
avocado ●
butter □
coconut ●
cream ●
ghee ●
margarine ●
vegetable oil □

LOW-STARCH VEGETABLES
arugula ●
asparagus ●
broccoli ●
Brussels sprouts ●
cabbage ●
cauliflower ●
celery ●
Chinese cabbage ●
collard ●
cucumber ●
eggplant ●
endive ●
escarole ●
garlic ●
green beans ●
kale ●
kohlrabi ●
leek ●
lettuce ●
lotus root ●
mushroom ●
mustard green ●
okra ●
onion ●
parsley ●
pepper ●
radish ●
scallion ●
sorrel ●
spinach ●
sprouts ●
summer squash ●
Swiss chard ●
turnip ●
turnip green ●
watercress ●
zucchini ●

HIGH-STARCH VEGETABLES
artichoke ●
beet ●
carrot ●
chestnut ●
corn ●
lima bean ●
parsnip ●
pea ●
potato ●
pumpkin ●
winter squash ●
yam ●

GRAIN PRODUCTS (STARCH)
amaranth ●
barley ●
buckwheat ●
millet ●
quinoa ●
kamut ●
kasha ●
oats ●
rice ●
rye ●
spelt ●
triticale ●
wheat ●

SUGARS
barley malt ●
brown sugar ●
honey ●
maple syrup ●
rice syrup ●
stevia ●
Sucanat ●
turbinado ●
white bread ●
white sugar ●

ACID FRUITS
grapefruit ◆
kiwi ◆
kumquat ◆
lemon ◆
lime ◆
orange ◆
pineapple ◆
strawberry ◆
tomato ◆

SUB ACID FRUITS
apple ●
apricot ●
blackberry ●
blueberry ●
cherry ●
grape ●
mango ●
nectarine ●
papaya ●
peach ●
pear ●
plum ●
raspberry ●
tangerine ●

SWEET FRUITS
banana ●
currant ●
date ●
fig ●
raisin ●

MELONS
cantaloupe ●
casaba ●
Christmas ●
honeydew ●
musk ●
watermelon ●

MISCELLANEOUS
fruit preserve ●
sugar-free jam ●
vinegar ●

Key
● Alkaline Foods—eat 4 for each 1 acid food
● Acid Foods—eat 1 for each 4 alkaline foods
□ Neutral Foods—remain neutral only when your pH is stable
◆ Acid Foods that convert to alkaline only when your pH is stable

Whole Health Food Classification Chart

To perform a food energy testing session using the EMT pass/fail test technique, the practitioner need only call out each food listed on the chart by name, while simultaneously pass/fail testing the subject's arm strength. *Practitioners must make sure to place their nondominant index finger directly on the subject's thyroid gland (at the base of the throat), while simultaneously calling out the name of each food being muscle tested.* This will maintain both partners' attention on the subject's thyroid gland, thus concentrating their intention to discover which foods support and which foods sabotage the subject's energetic metabolism.

There are many different ways to perform food energy muscle testing. The EMT system also includes procedures in which the practitioner can hold either real foods or homeopathic food vials to the throat of the subject. This approach would likely feel more comfortable to someone who's mechanistically biased, but it's not necessary. *If properly tuned*, you'll obtain the same accurate results by simply calling out the names of the foods you're looking to test the subject for. If not, simply retune!

When the partners have finished preparing and are in testing position, the practitioner can begin calling out the listed test foods one at a time. As each food is called out, the practitioner should gently and fluidly push at the wrist of the subject's outstretched arm, in order to test the subject's energy resistance after having audibly registered the food's name.

If the subject's arm weakens and fails at the sound of any food that the practitioner calls out, this indicates a failed food energy test. Remember, all pass and fail test results discovered while the practitioner's nondominant index finger lies on the subject's thyroid gland are representative of those foods that either help or hamper the subject's weight loss metabolism. Practitioners must make sure to immediately cross out any food that fails from the subject's Whole Health Food Classification Chart. Slowly run down the entire food list, carefully testing one food at a time while crossing out the failed foods. Once the pass/fail procedure is completed for the food energy test, practitioner and subject should then go on to perform EMT pulse testing.

Pulse testing enables partners to identify, in a quantifiable way, those foods that will best support or most harm the subject's prospects for metabolic weight loss efficiency. Far beyond simply revealing which foods are best and worst for the subject's thyroid metabolism, pulse testing provides quantifiable details as to just how good or bad a given food is.

The EMT pulse testing procedure begins with the practitioner stating aloud that he or she is about to pulse test positive foods on a scale from plus 1 to plus 10, and negative foods from minus 1 to minus 10. The practitioner must call out each food on the classification chart as he or she tests the subject's tolerance to the mention of each food. Some will pass and some will fail.

The subject's food energy responses will show precisely how positive or negative each food is for his or her thyroid gland (metabolism). The number of pulses are measured in relative numbers from plus 1 to plus 10 for positive foods (foods that passed in the pass/fail procedure), and from minus 1 to minus 10 for negative foods (foods that failed in the pass/fail procedure), with 1 representing the lowest and 10 representing the highest relative number. In pulse testing, the practitioner gently places his or her nondominant finger on the subject's thyroid, states aloud the name of a food, and pushes down the arm of the subject. A positive food that takes between plus 7 and plus 10 pushes before the arm falls is a strong result, meaning the named food is among the best possible metabolic support foods for that subject. A negative food that takes between minus 7 and minus 10 pushes is also a strong result, but in the opposite direction, meaning that that food is among the worst possible metabolically sabotaging foods for the subject.

Practitioners must be careful to remain sharply attuned to the exact count when the subject's arm falls. Any food that results in a positive muscle test between a pulse count of plus 7 and plus 10 should be considered an energetically optimal metabolic food for that subject. If the subject's arm weakens and falls at a pulse count between minus 1 and minus 10, whatever food was called out should be considered an energy-depleting food for the subject. All foods that pulse between plus 6 and minus 10 should be avoided.

Once practitioner and subject have completed all EMT pass/fail and pulse testing procedures, they're now prepared to map out the subject's Whole Health Diet plan. Now the subject isn't merely being given some generic weight loss diet. Instead, he or she is creating an energetically customized nutritional plan specifically designed to support his or her thyroid for maximum metabolic efficiency. Practitioners and subjects are encouraged to work hard at mastering these EMT protocols. These protocols make the WHD the only diet plan in the world that is energetically customized. It is also advisable to retest at least once a month, if not once a week, in order to keep up with the ever-changing energies that play such a significant role in a person's ever-changing metabolism and weight loss.

4. CUSTOMIZED MEAL PLAN TESTING

The customized meal plan testing provides subjects with their very own Acutrition diet. Where pass/fail and pulse testing enable them to identify their specific optimal metabolic foods, customized meal plan testing provides the finer details regarding the exact proper amounts to be taken throughout the day. Once again, this is a muscle testing procedure that taps into both the practitioner's and the subject's energy guidance system (EGS) for the answers.

The two partners will require a Whole Health meal plan chart for this exercise.

Customized meal plan testing combines both the EMT pass/fail and pulse testing techniques. The practitioner and subject begin with the EMT positioning and pass/fail testing, followed by pulse testing and tuning. They then pass/fail test for the subject's optimal daily meal format, one meal at a time, beginning with breakfast and moving on to morning snack, lunch, afternoon snack, dinner, and evening snack. Practitioners should simply name each meal as they muscle test the subject. Assuming that the subject's arm remains strong for the word "breakfast," the practitioner should then state aloud the words "protein," "vegetables," "fruits," and "high-starch carbohydrates" one at a time, while simultaneously testing the subject's strength for each. This pass/fail test reveals which specific food category is best for the subject's breakfast meal. Next, they will do pulse testing on amounts for breakfast: the practitioner audibly calls out amounts in ounces for whichever foods passed for breakfast while administering the pulse testing technique. For example, if protein passed for breakfast, the practitioner would call out amounts—for example, "three ounces," followed by a strength test; "four ounces," followed by a second strength test; and so on. Remember to keep up with your charting notes immediately following each test response. Test all meals, foods, and amounts until the meal plan is completed. Customized meal plan testing should be repeated at least once a month and as frequently as once a week, if time allows.

These quantum energy protocols are what separate the WHD from every other diet. First of all, every other diet obtains its information from the world in the form of "experts," authors, and theorists. The WHD's source of information is the stream of higher consciousness—the innate wellspring of wisdom that resides within each dieter. By mastering the WHD's innovative protocols, dieters will ultimately gain open access to their own inherent intelligence. In essence, by tuning dieters in to their "source power," the WHD awakens in them their inborn expertise. Moreover, it empowers dieters with the ability to customize their own personalized diet and to update their plan so that they may keep abreast of their ever-changing energy needs.

5. RAW VERSUS COOKED FOOD TEST

There is an ongoing debate as to whether raw or cooked food is nutritionally superior. Raw food advocates would remind us that uncooked foods contain a higher concentration of living enzymes and fiber. They insist that the more natural and undisturbed a food is, the healthier it is. They often point to the fact that by cooking food, you run the risk of destroying its vital enzymes. On the other hand there are those experts who posit that cooked, warm foods lend support to digestion in a different way. Many believe that when foods are served warm, they fortify spleen, stomach, lymph, and immune energies via thermogenic transference. Once again, the WHD reminds us that one size does not fit all. We are all constitutionally unique. Those constitutional types that suffer from constant colds, flu, and allergies are inclined to do better with warm, cooked foods. Those constitutional types that suffer from hypertension and heart disease are more inclined to do better with cold, raw foods. That said, debates such as this can be easily resolved. EMT pass/fail testing is an exceptional way to arrive at an energetically individualized conclusion. The subject holds up his or her arm and resists, as described earlier for pass/fail testing, while the practitioner gently presses it down and audibly states the words "warm, cooked food." Next, he or she repeats the same strength test as the practitioner says, "cold, raw food." They will discover one of three results. The subject will pass only for cooked, only for raw, or for both. If the subject passes both the cooked and the raw food tests, then practitioner and subject should pulse test both options to see which option scores a higher number between 1 and 10.

Not only will this simple test resolve a great debate, but, more important, it will provide subjects with yet another dietary articulation to further maximize their metabolism.

6. NUTRITIONAL SUPPLEMENT TESTING

Having completed their thyroid and food testing procedures, practitioner and subject should then go on to perform EMT nutritional supplement testing. Before beginning this procedure, redraw or photocopy the chart on the next page, which lists the supplements recognized by the WHD as proven agents that provide support for hypothyroidism (underactive thyroid).

To begin, the partners assume proper EMT positioning. Then the practitioner should perform pass/fail testing on the subject for each supplement listed. The pass/fail test should be immediately followed by pulse testing. This is where the practitioner pulse tests the subject's nutritional supplement response from 1 to 10, but only for those supplements that elicited a positive result

SUPPLEMENT	POTENCY	DOSE	FREQUENCY	DURATION
Selenomethionine (200 mcg capsule)				
Zinc gluconate (50 mg tablet)				
Kelp (250 mcg tablet)				
L-tyrosine (500 mg capsule)				
Pyridoxal 5'-phosphate (50 mg capsule)				
B complex (50 mg capsule)				
Floravital liquid (1 teaspoon)				

during the pass/fail testing. The practitioner must announce out loud the intention to test positive supplements in degrees of 1 to 10, and then commence. The subject is advised to take only those nutritional supplements that pulse test between a plus 8 and a plus 10.

Finally, the partners are ready to pass/fail test the subject's nutritional supplements for potency, dose, frequency, and duration—you know the right supplements to take; now it's time to figure out exactly how to take them. Let's begin by using selenomethionine as an example. The practitioner first calls out the above listed baseline potencies and then tests the subject's strength for baseline and incrementally higher dose callouts. I find that the highest potency produces a naturally strong muscle response. Once the test is completed, you will have discovered the subject's most efficient supplement dosage.

In the same pass/fail fashion, practitioners should call out doses, or the number of times per day the subject should take selenomethionine. The practitioner should call out "once a day" followed by a strength test, then "twice a day," and so on, until the arm drops. It's important to find the highest number of times a day that produces a strong muscle response. This represents the proper dose.

Next, the two are ready to test for frequency, or the number of days per week the selenomethionine is to be taken. The practitioner muscle tests the subject (pass/fail) while simultaneously calling out "one day per week," "two days per week," and so on for each supplement, until arriving at the most days per week that renders a strong muscle response. This represents the optimal frequency for taking each supplement.

Finally, partners test for duration, or the length of time the subject is to remain on a given nutritional supplement. As before, the practitioner will simultaneously strength test the subject (pass/fail) while stating "one week," "two weeks," "three weeks," "one month," and so on, until concluding with the highest number of weeks that produces a strong muscle response. This procedure represents duration. If partners wish to test one step further, they may check for duration cycles. Supplement plans often have a duration period that manifests in cycles. In other words, entire protocols can sometimes test positively for one month or so, but the subject may require a week or two off before beginning a new cycle. So the duration cycle may last for, say, three months followed by a two-week rest period. This allows the body to get caught up with absorption of weak supplement saturation. These respites often prove to be helpful when it comes to balancing metabolism.

The WHD 333 Rotation Diet and Recipe Plan

There is a direct connection between food and disease. For more than three decades, I've helped a great many people overcome disease through nutritional therapy. In most cases, these remarkable recoveries were the result of my "addition through subtraction" approach to nutrition, which calls for the elimination of toxic, inflammatory, allergenic, and *poorly rotated foods*. I'm not just talking about fat-laden, irradiated, sugary, fermented, allergenic foods. I'm also talking about static diets. Eating clean, healthy food—but failing to rotate those foods—can spell disaster when it comes to triggering genetic disease expressions.

Genes represent the molecular units of our hereditary blueprint. They are the archives that retain the vital instructions for our cellular construction, which produces our many traits and is responsible for repairing damage to our bodies. Our genetic archives are passed on to our offspring. We have thirty thousand genes that define our fixed material blueprint, or genetic code. I say "fixed" because our genes cannot change more than one-tenth of 1 percent every 250 generations. Our genetic code may be fixed, but the way our genes behave, or express themselves, is mutable.

You see, genes are like a light switch that can turn on and off. Each gene has what is called a "promoter" that, if prompted, can turn good or bad outcomes on or off in an instant. Research has proven that good genes are turned on and bad genes are silenced, by things like a clean, healthy, and properly rotated diet. By the same token, diseases and health conditions such as obesity are more often than not the result of bad genes switched on by toxic, allergenic, and poorly rotated meal plans. To get and maintain the WHD edge, you must avoid toxic, inflammatory, allergenic foods—and *rotate your diet*!

Assuming at this point that you've improved your food safety and quality and completed your entire battery of EMT screening, the next step is to learn how to prepare your meals and to set up the WHD 333 Plan. This plan provides you with breakfast, lunch, and dinner recipes designed to support a three-day, hypoallergenic, anti-inflammatory rotation diet. It also includes two healthy snacks per day.

The three-day rotation diet concept is really quite simple. Let's say you eat egg whites for breakfast on Monday. You would then have to avoid egg whites on Tuesday, Wednesday, and Thursday, making sure not to repeat them as a breakfast option until Friday. This cycling procedure would be similarly repeated for all proteins, low-starch vegetables, high-starch carbohydrates, and fruits in each meal. And though the WHD's EMT food allergy testing and the meal plan enable you to pinpoint and avoid the most allergenic foods, the three-day rotation diet will help to keep you from experiencing recurring food allergies.

The two most important things to know about food intolerances are these: foods that the body doesn't recognize (allergens) are inflammatory, and safe foods that are not rotated *become* inflammatory. In other words, let's assume that after having tested positive for egg whites, you decided to eat them every morning for a week straight—you'd likely develop an intolerance to them. Hardly a day goes by when I don't see a patient who tells me he or she was doing exceptionally well, staying symptom-free, and feeling great the first month of the diet, only to have symptoms return due to a lack of dietary rotation. Virtually all of these people return to an optimal state of wellness once they get solidly positioned into a three-day rotation. This three-day diet rotation is important for keeping the body, digestive system, and metabolism in tip-top condition.

The WHD 333 Recipes

It's important to remember that all foods and ingredients in the WHD's recipes must be USDA organic, free range, and wild.

Day 1 ☙ Breakfast:
EGG WHITE VEGGIE SCRAMBLE

This deliciously satisfying, low-fat, low-cholesterol, high-protein breakfast will start your day off with a calorie-burning boost! Egg whites are rich in the mineral selenium, which is known to support the thyroid's calorie-burning T4 hormone. They are also high in riboflavin (vitamin B$_2$), which plays a key role in the metabolism of fats.

> **2 tablespoons olive oil**
> **½ medium Vidalia onion, diced**
> **¾ cup diced red bell pepper**
> **1 clove garlic, minced**
> **2½ cups spinach leaves**
> **6–8 egg whites**
> **2 tablespoons coconut milk**

- Place olive oil in a sauté pan and set to low-medium heat.
- Add onions, peppers, garlic, and spinach to pan and sauté on low-medium heat until spinach shrinks down and onions become golden.

- In a bowl, place egg whites and coconut milk and whisk for twenty seconds. Pour into pan.
- Scramble until eggs are cooked to your liking.

SERVES FIVE.

Day 1 ✑ Lunch:
HI-PRO SALAD

This refreshing, nutritious salad provides sufficient protein to help keep your midday metabolism active. It also delivers an abundance of vitamins, minerals, and bowel-healthy insoluble fiber to support the upper and lower intestinal tracts.

4 cups mixed greens
½ small red/purple onion, thinly sliced
1 medium tomato, cut into wedges
1 medium cucumber, thinly sliced
8 ounces sliced turkey breast
4 tablespoons extra-virgin olive oil
Juice of 1 large lemon
3 tablespoons pure water
A dash each of thyme, rosemary, sage, and dill

- In two separate serving bowls, evenly divide the mixed greens, onion, tomato, cucumber, and turkey.
- In a teacup, blend the olive oil, lemon juice, water, and herbs.
- Add equal parts dressing to each bowl.

SERVES TWO.

Day 1 ❧ Dinner:
IMMUNE BOOSTER TURKEY BURGER *with asparagus*

This dinner recipe contains some of the spices known to be highest in antioxidants. According to recent USDA studies, turmeric, cumin, rosemary, and sweet basil are among the spices with the highest ORAC value, or oxygen radical absorbance capacity, as discussed earlier. The spices used in the Immune Booster Turkey Burger are estimated to have ten to twenty times more antioxidant power than the highest foods!

10 ounces 92% lean ground turkey
2 scallions, thinly sliced
½ clove garlic, minced
A dash each of turmeric, cumin, rosemary, marjoram, and sage
1 tablespoon coconut spread
A dash of sweet basil
¼ cup pure water
12 spears of asparagus
1 slice yeast-free, gluten-free oat bread

- Start water in the bottom of a steamer for the asparagus.
- In a bowl, blend the ground turkey with the scallions, garlic, turmeric, cumin, rosemary, marjoram, and sage. Form the mix into two equal-size patties.
- Place the coconut spread in a sauté pan and set to low-medium heat.
- Place the patties in pan and sprinkle a dash of sweet basil on top.
- Add the water to pan and cover with lid.

- Cook, covered, on low-medium heat for fifteen minutes on one side only. Because the burger is covered, it need not be flipped.
- While the burgers cook, steam asparagus until tender, about twelve minutes.
- Serve each burger on a slice of bread, with asparagus on the side.

SERVES TWO.

Day 2 ⁓ Breakfast:
CHICKEN BREAKFAST SAUSAGE SPECIAL *with grapefruit*

Breakfast protein is the single most important element of effective weight loss. Unlike typical, high-starch-carbohydrate breakfasts, this tasty high-protein option supports sustained calorie-burning action. According to a study recently published in the American Journal of Clinical Nutrition, *by ensuring that our dietary protein intake accounts for at least 30 percent of our total daily calories, we markedly decrease appetite and increase our prospects for weight loss. Studies have also shown grapefruit to be a powerful appetite suppressant!*

3 organic chicken breakfast sausages

A dash of garlic powder

1 grapefruit

- Preheat toaster oven to 350 degrees for eight minutes.
- Place sausages on a toaster oven tray and sprinkle with garlic powder.
- Bake for fifteen minutes.
- Serve with grapefruit.

SERVES ONE.

Day 2 ☙ Lunch:
SOUTHWEST CHICKEN AND BABY SPINACH SALAD

Capsaicin is the active thermogenic (heat-generating) agent in chili peppers. According to recent animal studies, capsaicin boosts metabolism and activates weight loss. As an added bonus, the folic acid in the spinach and ellagitannins in the pomegranate juice offer powerful anti-inflammatory support.

3 tablespoons grape-seed oil, divided

2 tablespoons pure water

10 ounces boneless, skinless chicken breast, split in half

¼ teaspoon chili powder

4 cups baby spinach leaves

¼ cup concentrated pomegranate juice

¼ cup pure water

- In a skillet place 1½ tablespoons of the grape-seed oil and the 2 tablespoons water.
- Coat chicken with chili powder and place in skillet.
- Cover skillet and cook for 15 minutes, checking occasionally.
- When chicken is done, cool for handling and slice into strips.
- Divide the baby spinach leaves into two salad bowls.
- In a teacup, blend dressing: the remaining 1½ tablespoons of grape-seed oil, the pomegranate juice, and the ¼ cup water.
- Dress each salad with equal parts dressing.
- Place chicken strips over salads and serve.

SERVES TWO.

Day 2 ❧ Dinner:
MEDITERRANEAN WHITE SAUCE
WITH GROUND CHICKEN *with broccoli and rice pasta*

Researchers tell us that oregano may be helpful for stubborn weight loss problems. A new animal study indicates that a powerful antioxidant called carvacral in oregano has been found to offset diet-induced obesity by neutralizing inflammation and modulating gene expression. In addition, according to researchers in the Netherlands, grape-seed oil has been shown to reduce calorie intake by 4 percent over a twenty-four-hour period. Researchers in Spain have found the oil to markedly improve insulin efficiency.

6 ounces rice pasta

3 tablespoons grape-seed oil, divided

2 celery stalks, diced

⅓ yellow bell pepper, diced

⅓ orange bell pepper, diced

1 medium plum tomato, diced

½ clove garlic, minced

1 tablespoon each of fresh oregano, parsley, marjoram, and sage

10 ounces 92% lean ground chicken breast

10 ounces free-range, organic, low-sodium chicken broth

½ cup pure water

■ Bring 2½ quarts water and the broth to full boil. Add rice pasta and boil nine to eleven minutes, stirring occasionally. Drain pasta in colander and return to same pan. Stir in 1 tablespoon of the grape-seed oil.

- While pasta cooks, oil skillet with remaining 2 tablespoons of the grape-seed oil and set at low-medium heat.
- Add the vegetables to the skillet and sauté with the herbs.
- When the vegetables begin to soften, add the ground chicken.
- Cover pan with lid and cook for twenty minutes, stirring occasionally.

SERVES TWO.

Day 3 ᔆ Breakfast:
MARK'S SOY (OR SOY-FREE) SMOOTHIE

For those who are tolerant to soy, this healthy, flavorful smoothie provides a rich, creamy, calorie-burning, anti-inflammatory breakfast option. A number of studies have shown this antioxidant-rich, low-fat protein reduces appetite by helping one to feel fuller longer. While there may be some debate as to whether soy is a healthy or unhealthy food, it's important to remember the WHD represents a personalized diet system in which food tolerances are individually determined by Electromagnetic Muscle Testing. If it passes the test, enjoy with the soy! If it fails, enjoy with the substitute ingredients listed.

½ **cake silken tofu**

2 scoops pea protein powder

8 drops liquid stevia

Dash of cinnamon

4 drops pure vanilla extract

10 ounces plain soy milk (or coconut milk)

2 tablespoons ground flaxseeds

½ cup fresh or frozen blueberries

- Place ingredients in a blender and puree until smooth.

SERVES TWO.

Day 3 ✥ **Lunch:**
ARUGULA SOCKEYE SALAD

Salmon's high-quality protein and anti-inflammatory omega-3 fatty acids make it the perfect meal option to promote satiety and curb appetite. The high fiber, vitamin K, and folate concentrations in the arugula provide excellent satiety support.

4 cups arugula

Two 6-ounce cans wild sockeye salmon, drained

3 tablespoons organic canola oil, divided

Juice of 1 clementine

Dash each of basil, chervil, coriander, and watercress

- Divide arugula equally in two salad bowls.
- Place contents of one can of salmon in each bowl.
- Dress each salad with 1½ tablespoons of the canola oil and half of the clementine juice.
- Sprinkle the herbs over each salad.

SERVES TWO.

Day 3 ❧ Dinner:
WILD SEA SCALLOPS OVER QUINOA *with kale*

These sweet, high-protein ocean delights contain a high concentration of the mineral io-dine. This makes them a perfect nutritional support food for the metabolism, as iodine is essential for healthy thyroid gland function. They are also high in selenium, which sup-ports the thyroid's metabolic T4 hormone management. Also, a serving of kale contains approximately 10 percent of the recommended daily allowance of fiber, which makes it a good "feel full" food.

> 1 cup pure water
>
> ½ cup quinoa
>
> 4 cups kale
>
> ⅛ teaspoon finely ground black pepper
>
> ⅛ cup chopped fresh parsley, oregano, and basil
>
> 1 clove shallot, minced
>
> 8 large wild sea scallops (about 12 ounces)
>
> 2 tablespoons avocado oil

- In a medium saucepan, bring water to boil and add quinoa. Cover, reduce heat to low, and simmer approximately fifteen minutes.
- Remove the stems from the kale, place the leaves in the top of a steamer, and steam until tender, about five minutes.
- Sprinkle pepper, parsley, oregano, basil, and shallot over scallops.
- Heat avocado oil in large skillet on medium-high heat.

- Place scallops in pan and sauté for two and a half minutes on each side, or until browned and opaque.
- On each of two plates serve 4 scallops on a ¾ cup bed of quinoa, with kale alongside.

SERVES TWO.

WHD 333 Food Rotation Quick Reference Guide

Day 1

Breakfast: *Egg White Veggie Scramble*
Midmorning: One large apple
Lunch: *Hi-Pro Salad*
Midafternoon: Three stalks of celery with 3 tablespoons of sesame-free hummus
Dinner: *Immune Booster Turkey Burger*—with asparagus

Day 2

Breakfast: *Chicken Breakfast Sausage Special*—with grapefruit
Midmorning: One large nectarine
Lunch: *Southwest Chicken and Baby Spinach Salad*
Midafternoon: One large nectarine with ¼ cup unsalted pumpkin seeds
Dinner: *Mediterranean White Sauce with Ground Chicken*—with broccoli and rice pasta

Day 3

    Breakfast: *Mark's Soy (or Soy-Free) Smoothie*

    Midmorning: ½ cup papaya chunks

    Lunch: *Arugula Sockeye Salad*

    Midafternoon: ½ cup papaya chunks with ¼ cup unsalted dry-roasted
       soy nuts

    Dinner: *Wild Sea Scallops over Quinoa*—with kale

Mastering the Art of Cheating

The WHD teaches that one of the prerequisites of successful long-term dieting and permanent weight loss is "mastering the art of cheating." We must bear in mind that regardless of how disciplined and determined we may be to follow a well-designed health protocol, we are still mere mortals. Everything in the mortal world is governed by what I call the Inhale, Exhale Law. Not unlike a heartbeat, in which energy is drawn in and released, there is a natural physics to the cycling of all energy. It's what the ancient Chinese referred to as "the way of things." It's why so much of the world has adopted work and school schedules that are more active during the weekdays and less active on weekends. We can put only so much energy into something before requiring a relaxing of our efforts. One of the most important positions put forth by the WHD is its 85 Percent Rule.

The WHD's 85 Percent Rule says unequivocally that before getting started, the dieter must immediately strike any and all thoughts of following the diet 100 percent. Any dieter who entertains a vision of following a diet 100 percent is only ensuring that he or she will hit the wall harder. It's simple logic. It can be compared to holding your breath as long as you can. The longer you hold your breath, the deeper you'll gasp for air after running out. So, by admitting right up front that you are a mere mortal, and that you're destined to lose a battle from time to time, you will actually enable yourself to win the war. It's not about passing and failing. It's about employing a strategy that includes calculated cheating.

The WHD's 85 Percent Rule advocates cheating within reason—one day per week at one meal per week. This doesn't mean to suggest that one consume an inordinate amount of fried food, half a cake, a pint of ice cream, and a bottle of wine! Rather, it means consuming a standard 600-calorie entrée appearing on a menu in an average family restaurant, along with a splurge along the lines of two clear vodka beverages or one 300-calorie dessert. Remember to choose a restaurant that you enjoy and invite people you love. The focus should not be on the food alone. The focus should also be on the environment and the experience. This should be an occasion that you look forward to and work hard for. It should be a reward that you use to your advantage. If properly mastered, your 15 percent, calculated, once-a-week cheat can inspire remarkable long-term results.

I've instituted this plan both in my private counseling practice and in my corporate consulting programs for thousands of people over the past thirty-two years, and I can tell you firsthand that it has proven to be a real difference maker.

I'm always amazed at the looks on people's faces when I explain the WHD 85 Percent Rule to them. Many of them have been programmed to think in very dysfunctional all-or-nothing terms. Once again, it's a good time to remind ourselves about one of the important tenets of the WHD—balance! While there are a growing number of diet plans that tell us that we can cheat and still lose weight, the WHD 85 Percent Rule firmly asserts that in order for people to succeed at long-term dieting and permanent weight loss, they must first master the art of cheating.

CHAPTER 7

BALANCING METABOLISM WITH ENERGY MEDICINE

Wenchiech'u

In order to attain and maintain a healthy weight, one must have a vibrant metabolism. Having a vibrant metabolism requires an energetically balanced body. The ancient Chinese healing art of wenchiech'u is an exceptional way to balance the energies of the body. Wenchiech'u is a form of qigong, or energy mastery, that has been practiced in China for more than five thousand years. Over the millennia, Chinese practitioners have employed various forms of qigong for the purposes of balancing and strengthening organ systems. Translated, *wenchiech'u* means "thermogenesis," as its stimulating effect infuses the body with a flow of warm vitality.

There are two forms of wenchiech'u—contact and noncontact thermogenesis. The contact form is quite simple. A practitioner places the index finger of his or her dominant hand directly on the thyroid gland of the subject (at the front base of the neck). Next, the practitioner can either stimulate the subject's underactive thyroid gland by circling the index finger in a counterclockwise

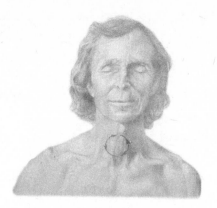

Thyroid Wenchiech'u

motion (imagining the subject as the clock, facing outward) or de-stimulate a subject's overactive thyroid gland by circling the index finger in a clockwise motion. So, counterclockwise motions generate a stimulating energy, and clockwise motions generate a de-stimulating energy. A powerful mental intention and a light touch directed in a circular motion is all it takes. This exercise should be practiced twice daily, morning and afternoon, for three minutes each time.

The WHD has added a wrinkle to wenchiech'u.

In order to help the practitioner determine whether the subject's thyroid is over- or underactive, the WHD recommends that every practitioner first administer diagnostic EMT pass/fail and pulse testing on the subject's thyroid. If the practitioner first establishes that the subject's thyroid fails a pass/fail test, then he or she should go on to pulse test the subject's thyroid with minus numbers from 1 to 10.

This pass/fail test, however, doesn't require the practitioner to call out any phrases, as the previous tests did. Instead, the light presence of the practitioner's finger on the subject's thyroid fulfills that function. The test result (the strength resistance of the subject's arm) will be either strong or weak. A strong response represents a pass. A weak response is a fail.

Following the pass/fail test, the pulse test reveals the degree of strength or weakness of the subject's thyroid. A minus 1 is not as deficient as a minus 2, and minus 10 would represent the lowest possible score. In any case, minus scores indicate an energetic hypothyroid response that calls for the administration of counterclockwise wenchiech'u for balancing.

On the other hand, assuming that the subject passes the pass/fail test, the subject and practitioner must then go on to pulse test for the potential of hyperthyroid. Positive pulse scores from 1 to 10 are considered healthy and balanced, with plus 10 reflecting the best possible energy score. If there appears to be exceedingly high resistance, then the practitioner should verbally call out the intention to test the subject's thyroid in unlimited numbers—if the subject's thyroid pulse test is higher than plus 10, such a score would indicate an energetic hyperthyroid response, necessitating the administration of clockwise wenchiech'u for balancing. Practitioners should also be prepared to retest the subject's thyroid after every twenty circular motions. This enables the practitioner to calibrate the subject's thyroid energy to an exact balance point. When combined with the EMT pass/fail and pulse testing techniques, wenchiech'u is a very powerful energy technique to help with thyroid balancing. Always remember to begin EMT with tuning to ensure greater accuracy.

The noncontact form of wenchiech'u can be successfully practiced by either the self or an experienced master. Once again, the key is to generate counter-clockwise spirals to stimulate, and clockwise spirals to de-stimulate. The main difference here is that the practitioner produces the spirals not with the touch of the index finger, but rather with the intention of his or her mind. Accomplished masters of wenchiech'u can also perform effective thermogenesis non-locally. That is, they can actually successfully engage wenchiech'u thyroid balancing at any distance. Though this may be difficult for some to believe, it's important to keep in mind that this healing technique has been successfully practiced for thousands of years. I can certainly attest to its validity from my thirty-two years and thousands of applications. Wenchiech'u is the most powerful vehicle for energy balancing that I know of. We must keep in mind that everything is energy, even thoughts. Thoughts that carry a powerful intention combined with intense concentration are among the most powerful manifestations of energy. Though they elude our five senses, thoughts are things.

Auricular Wenchiech'u

The WHD's auricular wenchiech'u was inspired by the healing art of auricular, or ear, acupuncture. Studies have clearly demonstrated that ear acupuncture can indeed help people to both reduce their body mass index and lose weight. A recent Korean study published in the British journal *Acupuncture in Medicine* found that when practitioners focused on five specific acupuncture points instead of just one, the results were markedly more noteworthy. Auricular acupuncture was pioneered in France in 1956 by Dr. Paul Nogier. Dr. Nogier envisioned the ear as a curled up fetus with its head pointing downward. He determined that the ear contains a full complement of acupuncture points that corresponded with all the body's major glands and organs, which he started mapping out in detail. He then began treating his patients by applying acupressure and acupuncture to the points on the ear associated with all the body's organs. Almost immediately, Nogier discovered that his patients were consistently experiencing positive results.[1]

In another study, reported in *Medical News Today*, researchers in Korea "Compared the efficacy of acupuncture treatments in helping obese patients lose weight, comparing the standard Korean five point treatment with acupuncture using a single point of stimulation. They also included a control group who were given a 'sham' treatment.

"In a randomized controlled clinical trial, 91 Koreans were recruited—16 men and 75 women—all of whom had a body mass index (BMI) equal to or greater than 23. None of the participants had received any other weight control treatments in the last 6 months.

"The participants were randomly divided into three groups, one group to receive the five point acupuncture treatment, another the one point acupuncture treatment and the third group, the control 'sham' treatment. . . .

"[O]f the participants who completed the trial, there were significant differences in results. At the midway point, there were already noticeable differences in BMI with the five point treatment group showing a 6.1% reduction, the one point group a 5.7% reduction, while the sham group showed no reduction at all. Both active treatment groups also showed weight loss."[2]

As with all wenchiech'u exercises, auricular wenchiech'u is a form of mental qigong, designed to stimulate the all-important acupuncture points on the ears by mentally projecting counterclockwise spirals from the mind's eye to the ears. With this particular metabolic stimulation exercise, one need not be concerned about targeting the five auricular acupuncture points. By transmitting thought energy to each ear in its entirety, one at a time, the five points will be sufficiently stimulated.

To perform auricular wenchiech'u, first make sure you're in a quiet, undisturbed place, then simply close your eyes and take three slow, deep, clearing breaths. Once you're settled and relaxed, begin to picture yourself transmitting stimulating counterclockwise-spiraling energy to your left ear first. That means the direction of the spin should go from the back of the left ear, in a circular arc over the top of the ear, to the front of the ear. Continue transmitting the counterclockwise-spiral energy for no more than a few minutes. Next, picture yourself transmitting stimulating counterclockwise-spiral energy to your right ear. The direction of this particular spin should go from the front of the right ear, in a circular arc over the top of the ear, to the back of the ear. Once again, no more than a few minutes are required here.

Auricular wenchiech'u combines elements of Korean acupuncture with Chinese qigong. This powerful exercise should be performed no more than once a day, preferably in the early morning.

Three-Point Acupressure Exercise

There are over one thousand acupuncture points on the human body. Each one has its own unique energetic properties, and when any given point is combined with other specifically designated points, the energy healing applications are infinite. The WHD's Three-Point Acupressure Exercise to balance metabolism emphasizes three very important acupuncture points: stomach 36, small intestine 19 (referred to as the "hunger point"), and conception vessel 6. This exercise should not be performed in late stages of pregnancy.

Weight gain from imbalanced metabolism is the result of a breakdown in the energy flow between the brain's regulatory hypothalamus, the metabolic endocrine system, and the liver. Studies have shown that acupuncture, acupressure, and qigong can help balance the leptin and ghrelin levels, thereby regulating appetite, cravings, and calorie-burning potential.

Stomach 36 is located on the front of the lower leg, one finger-length below the kneecap and one finger-width outward from the edge of the shinbone (the tibia). This point has a great many applications but has a specific affinity for tonifying poor digestion.

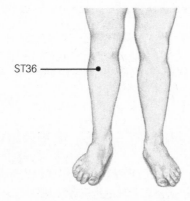

Stomach 36

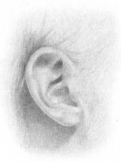

The Hunger Point

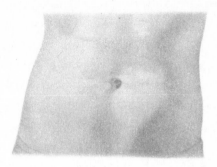

Conception Vessel 6

Small intestine 19, the "hunger point," is located on the front of the tragus (the prominence at the opening of the ear), in the center on the transitional fold. This point has been used for thousands of years to suppress appetite, stimulate metabolism, and improve digestion.

Conception vessel 6 is one of the most important acupuncture points in the human body. It is located 1¾ inches below the center of the umbilicus. This point stimulates the dormant energy of the body, thus increasing general metabolic output. It is also known to tonify the stomach energy and improve digestive efficiency.

Performing the Three-Point Acupressure Exercise is quite simple. First, find a quiet place to sit and relax for three to five minutes. Begin by clearing all existing oxygen from your lungs. Immediately follow the cleansing breath by taking a deep inhalation. Hold the breath for a count of four seconds, then release.

Now place your index finger directly on the stomach 36 point, applying moderate pressure. Keep your finger pressed down on the point for approximately thirty seconds. Next, pulse your finger up and down, slowly and repeatedly, alternating between shallow and deep pressure, for an additional thirty seconds. Finally, once again place your index finger directly on the point with moderate pressure for thirty seconds, then release. Next, follow the same directions for small intestine 19 and conception vessel 6, in that order.

The Three-Point Acupressure Exercise should be practiced once a day, preferably in the morning. Remember, do not perform this exercise in late stages of pregnancy.

Pranayama

Fat is composed of oxygen, hydrogen, and carbon. Oxygen ultimately circulates into fat cells, breaking them down and converting them into carbon dioxide and water. Blood then carries the carbon dioxide molecules into the lungs, where they can be released. The more oxygen our bodies generate, the more fat we'll incinerate. Metabolism is like a fire. Without oxygen, fire dies out. So weight loss has everything to do with the way we breathe.

Stress also plays a significant role in metabolism. It upsets the entire nervous system. Seventy percent of the nervous system runs through the digestive tract. Therefore, when stress is high, digestive efficiency is low. Moreover, when stress levels are elevated, hormones like cortisol, adrenaline, and ghrelin will also elevate, resulting in brain-driven patterns of uncontrolled overeating. So by consistently calming and balancing our nervous system, we will also keep our calorie-burning metabolism in better balance.

One of the most ancient forms of balancing, healing breath work is pranayama, or "yogic breathing." The word *pranayama* represents two Sanskrit words, *prana*, "breath," and *ayama*, "circulation." For our purposes in this book, we will focus on a pranayama exercise referred to as "circular breathing." It's quite simple, powerful, and effective.

Pranayamic circular breathing can be practiced anywhere, but is most effective in a quiet, comfortable, undisturbed setting. Begin by clearing your breath. By that, I mean emptying out all stale air as you prepare to take in fresh, energizing oxygen. Next, place your right thumb over your right nostril so that it's blocking your right nostril's ability to take in air. Then simply inhale through your left nostril for a slow count of four. Now, place your last two fingers over your left nostril. As you hold the breath in with both nostrils blocked, count slowly to four, continuing to hold the breath in. Then lift your right thumb at the right nostril and release the breath for a count of four. Return your right thumb to the right nostril so that both nostrils are again blocked, and hold the breath out for a slow count of four. This represents one complete pranayamic circular breathing cycle. Now you're prepared to begin the cycle again by inhaling through your left nostril for a slow count of four. Take the time to perform four complete cycles. Then, reverse the circular motion of your breathing by repeating this entire exercise in the opposite direction.

This pranayamic circular breathing exercise will immediately improve your metabolism by balancing your oxygenation and stress chemistries. It is recommended that you practice this exercise once daily.

Metabolic Homeopathy

Homeopathy is a system of medicine that treats subjects with highly diluted substances with the intention of activating the body's own natural, innate healing powers. The word "homeopathy" means "like cures like." Thus, the highly diluted substances that are used in homeopathic treatments are energetic agents that, in material form, are likely to cause the very symptoms that they're intended to heal. For example, the homeopathic remedy Allium cepa (red onion) would, for obvious reasons, be the perfect medicine for a condition known as epiphora—or watery eyes. Similar to vaccines that contain toxins, germs, and viruses, homeopathic medicines are derived from just about everything under the sun. The main difference between homeopathic and inoculation theory is that homeopathy dilutes its—dare I say "medicinal"?—toxic agents down to where there are no remaining material properties. When reading words like "belladonna" and "arsenic" on your homeopathic labels, you must keep in mind that nothing but energy remains therein. It's always a counterintuitive exercise to read a homeopathic label with the understanding that it's a safe medication that causes no serious side effects. For these are medicines prepared from toxic ingredients, designed to reverse symptoms by energetically creating a perfect match between illness and cure.

Established in 1796 by Samuel Hahnemann, homeopathy subscribes to the idea that disease is a phenomenon caused by states called miasms. Described as energetic states that predispose us to potential future illnesses, miasms may remain dormant for years and even generations, but eventually can flare up to cause chronic or acute illnesses. Viral or bacterial traits are contained within cells, which means a miasm is not necessarily disease but rather potential for disease. Dr. Hahnemann identified three inherited miasms:

1. Psoric—the mother of all disease; rhythmic imbalance between body and mind
2. Syphilitic/gonorrheal—sexual transmission with destructive effect on all tissues and bones
3. Sycotic—sexual transmission (particularly gonorrheal) causing deposits, congestion, and tumor formations; disorders are found in the pelvic and sexual areas as well as skin, digestive, respiratory, and urinary tract

The concept of miasms reveals the true holistic nature of homeopathy. There are believed to be thirty-eight thousand diseases occurring from one or more of the inherited miasms. Hahnemann was far ahead of his time. Today many credit him with being the father of both holistic and energy medicine in the West.

Homeopathic medicines are indeed energy based. Their mode of action generates subcellular vibratory frequencies. Homeopathy is etheric medicine—it operates beyond the physical frequency and has a magnetic presence that vibrates far beyond light velocity. "Homeopathic remedies represent an alternative evolutionary pathway in the application of medicinal plant therapies," says physician and researcher Richard Gerber. "Where pharmacologists chose to isolate single, active molecular agents from herbs, homeopaths worked with the vibrational essence of the whole plant substance. The homeopathic preparation process liberates from the plants the subtle energetic qualities to charge water, from which they are then transferred to milk sugar tablets for individualized dosage. Thus homeopathic remedies differ from pharmacologic agents in that they are 'etherealized' medicines."[3] Etherealized medicines, to this day, remain highly controversial.

The mechanistic Western mentality is generally at a distinct disadvantage when it comes to understanding the quantum nature of such medicine. Nonetheless, homeopathy remains popular worldwide, especially in Europe, where it boasts one hundred million regular users. As many as 44 percent of Dutch doctors say they rely upon homeopathy as a primary medicine.[4] In India, according to Dana Ullman, a frequent writer on homeopathy, "Over 100 million people depend solely on this form of medical care." Ullman further cites a 2007 A. C. Neilsen survey that says 62 percent of them say they "have never tried conventional medicines," and 82 percent say they "would not switch to conventional treatments."[5]

Here in the United States, homeopathic medicines are regulated by the U.S. FDA and are readily available in health food stores and pharmacy chains. There have been a number of interesting studies in recent years, with some that have drawn the attention of the American public.

Supported by numerous clinical trials, a diet using the homeopathic preparation of human chorionic gonadotropin (hCG) has been shown to activate metabolism by increasing anabolic hormone levels, while significantly reducing appetite. This diet imposes caloric restrictions of 500 to 800 calories per day for extended periods of time, while supplementing with homeopathic drops of human chorionic gonadotropin hormone. The homeopathic drops are said to signal the hypothalamus gland to release fat. According to one preliminary study, hundreds of patients were clinically tested via blood, EKGs, and electrolytes. Positive results were noted. These preliminary studies were followed up with four randomized, double-blind, placebo-controlled trials. When the hCG group was compared with the placebo group, there were significant differences in subjects' fat-to-muscle ratio. Both the placebo group and the hCG group lost an average of thirteen to fifteen pounds per month during the study, but the hCG group lost only two pounds of muscle, while the placebo group lost five pounds of muscle.[6] The hCG homeopathic program is a prescription program. There are also a number of inexpensive, readily available, over-the-counter homeopathic medicines that are safe and effective at supporting weight loss.

Keep in mind that homeopathy can support weight loss only when it accompanies a sound dietary plan. It's not likely that one could lose weight with homeopathy alone. That said, below are the WHD's five favorite homeopathic medicines to assist with weight loss.

1. Calcarea carbonica (carbonate of lime) is principally indicated for belly fat and low metabolism. It's considered a preeminent homeopathic remedy for chronic weight gain and obesity and is indicated for those who have a tendency to perspire profusely, especially around the head, or have chronic constipation, an underactive pituitary, hypothyroidism, and intolerance to cold air.

2. Nux vomica (poison nut) is a great homeopathic polychrest medicine that might prove helpful for those overweight, sedentary types who suffer from

severe chronic constipation and chills. Nux vomica is indicated for those people drawn to rich, fatty foods, alcoholic beverages, and caffeine, who may also tend to be highly stressed, overactive, nervous, and irritable. This homeopathic remedy is also best for those who commonly suffer from inflammatory stress headaches.

3. Ignatia amara (St. Ignatius bean) is an exceptional medicine for aiding weight loss in those who also experience deep, overwhelming emotion—especially sadness and chronic depression. Those most likely to benefit from Ignatia are inclined to cycle between mania and depression. These emotional vicissitudes are often accompanied by spikes in appetite that result in emotional binge eating.

4. Fucus vesiculosus (sea kelp), in its potentized form (see next page), fortifies the thyroid gland—improving its ability to produce and absorb metabolism-stimulating thyroid hormone. Those who suffer from chronic constipation and a sensation of pressure around the head are likely to do very well with this remedy.

5. Antimonium crudum (black sulphide of antimony) increases metabolism, improves digestion, and eliminates sluggishness. This medicine is indicated where there is a history of poor assimilation, indigestion, bloating, and gas. The patient best suited for Antimonium vacillates between sentimental and angry moods and frequently suffers from nausea, nosebleeds, headaches, and hair loss.

Unlike material medicines, homeopathic medicines are energy based—therefore, the more they are diluted, the higher their potency. This is difficult for most mechanistic minds to grasp. I like to think of it in terms of a drawstring effect, in which material medicine is on one side and energy medicine is on the other. If both medicines are diluted, the material medicine will get weaker, but the energy medicine will get stronger. The reason for this is that only matter can be diluted, and as it is, energy becomes more activated.

Homeopathy engages a process known as potentization, in which the medicinal agents are diluted with distilled water and then vigorously shaken to stir up the vital energies contained within the diluted substance. Samuel Hahnemann created several potency scales for medicinal dilution, each signified in Roman numerals. The three most common potency scales are: X, which represents ten dilutions; C, which stands for one hundred dilutions; and M, representing one thousand dilutions. Each of these potency scales is then further broken down to numbers of six, twelve, and thirty. Therefore, the potency of 6X (six times ten) would signify sixty dilutions, and a potency of 30C (thirty times one hundred) would represent three thousand dilutions. Keep in mind, the more material diluting, the higher the energetic potency. Hahnemann himself generally advocated 30C dilutions. Many experts are of the opinion that the higher the homeopathic potency, the greater the likelihood of the medicine reaching deeper into the holistic aspects of body, mind, and spirit. Anyone considering working with the previously mentioned homeopathic medicines might do well to purchase 30C potency. Homeopathic medicines at 30C potency are readily available, over the counter, at most neighborhood health stores. As far as dosing goes, it's generally recommended to dissolve three or four pellets under the tongue, three times a day, seven days a week, for at least one month.

For more detailed information, you should read up on any remedy in the Homeopathic Materia Medica, typically available at most health food stores and online. While homeopathic medicines are considered very safe for general use, it's a good idea to consider consulting with a professional homeopath.

Bach Flower Essences

Edward Bach was an early-twentieth-century British orthodox medical practitioner who took homeopathy to another level. It was said that during his youth, he displayed an abiding love of nature and was often seen wandering about the rural countryside near his home, enjoying the splendor and beauty of the indigenous flowering botanicals. Even at that time, he was noted for his uncommon powers of intuition, and word soon spread of his mystical ability to communicate with the flowers and herbs of the neighboring countryside.

Later in life, as a physician in London, he traveled to the countryside as much as possible for the love of his life—botany. He was afraid that the allure of the countryside botanicals would prove too much of a distraction from the medical career to which he was so deeply committed. From 1914 until nearly 1919, Bach continued to study botany and maintain a practice of orthodox medicine. His further study of health and disease eventually inspired him to delve into homeopathy. During these years, he performed a great deal of original research in these two divergent fields of medicine. He gave many lectures and contributed noteworthy articles in medical journals on the findings of his research. Ultimately, the homeopathic medical establishment held him in the highest regard.

Over time, Bach integrated the disciplines of orthodox medicine, homeopathy, and botany, as he began studying the medicinal potentials of flowering botanicals. From the fall of 1928 through the late summer of 1936, Edward Bach collected flowering plants from the English and Welsh countryside. In accordance with the treatises of homeopathy, he prepared medicinal tinctures from these flowers and developed meticulous preparation methods, which demanded specific exposure to both the sun and the moon. His intuition was said to be his chief guiding influence, as he seemed to somehow know that these flowering essences and their magnetic resonance with the sun and moon would have a profound impact on the subtle energies of other living beings.

Bach was far ahead of his time in understanding the relationship between stress and disease. In the minds of many, he is the Western world's pioneer of mind-body medicine. In his book *The Twelve Healers and Other Remedies*, he wrote, "Thus, behind all disease lie our fears, our anxieties, our greed, our likes and dislikes. Let us seek these out and heal them, and with the healing of them will go the disease from which we suffer."[7] Bach clearly understood that human emotion generates energetic powers, which ultimately manifest in the material realm as physical symptoms and disease.

Today, Bach's healing flower essences are extracted from shrubs, trees, and wildflowers from locations around the world. Numbering thirty-eight in all, each is believed to bring about a different vibrational healing influence to the patient, capable of balancing one's energy from the subtlest thought and emotional levels to the physical somatic levels. Ingested, the flower essence remedies are first absorbed in the blood and are then transported to the central nervous system. It is there where they interact with the vibrational imbalances, prior to gaining entry into the body's energy pathways.

Where much of the stress of weight gain and weight loss is rooted in emotion, the Bach Flower Remedies represent subtle but effective balancing energy medicine options.

The remedies may be orally ingested, added to the bath, massaged into tissues, or spritzed near the body in order to affect the electromagnetic field. There are a number of Bach Materia Medicas—lists of the remedies along with their uses—available at health stores and bookstores to help you decide which remedies are best for you.

Here's the WHD's abbreviated Materia Medica:

1. Rock Rose—For panic, hysteria, and fear of loss of control.
2. Mimulus—For fear within the realm of known worldly circumstances.
3. Cherry Plum—For uncontrollable, obsessive panic.
4. Aspen—For psychological fears of the unknown, and free-floating anxiety.
5. Red Chestnut—For obsessive worry about the well-being of others.
6. Cerato—For self-doubt, negative self-image, and lack of self-confidence.
7. Scleranthus—For indecisiveness, lack of concentration, and ADHD-like symptoms.
8. Gentian—For discouragement, loss of faith, and hopelessness.
9. Gorse—For grief, sadness, and deep despair.
10. Hornbeam—For overwhelming physical fatigue, and inability to face the burdens of the day.

11. Wild Oat—For despondency resulting from unfulfilled desires.

12. Clematis—For absentmindedness, drowsiness, and lack of interest in the present. Good for learning disabilities and ADD.

13. Honeysuckle—For nostalgic heartache and homesickness. For the torment of being stuck in the past.

14. Wild Rose—For apathy and lack of life spark; utter discouragement and despondency.

15. Olive—For complete physical and mental exhaustion; feeling run-down from long, depleting ordeals.

16. White Chestnut—For recurring, obsessive-compulsive thought patterns that cycle on without resolution.

17. Mustard—For depression or gloom that comes on suddenly without any apparent cause or origin.

18. Chestnut Bud—For those who fail to learn from experience.

19. Water Violet—For those whose pride forces them to withdraw to bear their trials alone.

20. Impatiens—For those who are too impulsive to exercise forbearance. For impatience.

21. Heather—For those who suffer from nervous constitutions and cannot bear to be left alone with their pain.

22. Agrimony—For those who show the world a bold face as a disguise for their inner torment.

23. Centaury—For those who are timid, weak willed, and easily dominated by more forceful personalities.

24. Walnut—For those who need protection from outside influences during

times of vulnerability. For grounding during times of transformation. Helps one to move on.

25. Holly—For any highly charged negative emotional state, including bitterness, anger, rage, or frustration.
26. Larch—For deeply negative expectations and faithless doubt.
27. Pine—For guilt, shame, and self-reproach. For timid souls, lacking in self-esteem, who are self-critical and readily accepting of blame.
28. Elm—For those who, while capable, feel they lack endurance to face the magnitude and responsibility of their tasks.
29. Sweet Chestnut—For times of deep despair, when one is at the outer limits of one's psychic endurance. This is the preeminent remedy for "the dark night of the soul."
30. Star of Bethlehem—For the overwhelming effects of any sudden, unexpected, shocking experience.
31. Willow—For resentment and blame. For those who fail to accept responsibility for their own life lessons.
32. Oak—For mental and emotional stamina in the face of recurring setbacks.
33. Crab Apple—For the cleansing of shame and the detoxification of self-contempt.
34. Chicory—For insecurity and addiction to control, safety, and predictability.
35. Vervain—For strong-opinioned, domineering personalities who overbearingly force their ideology on others.
36. Vine—For those ruthless people who feel constantly driven to dominate others.

37. Beech—For those critical, judgmental, intolerant personalities, who are constantly annoyed at the idiosyncratic ways of others.

38. Rock Water—For repressed, self-restricted, obsessive types, who feel shamefully undeserving and often deny themselves the simple pleasures of life.

Rescue Remedy is a mixture that combines impatiens, clematis, rock rose, cherry plum, and star of bethlehem. This remedy is designed specifically for the emotional and psychological disturbances that may occur during times of emergency.

Typically, the Bach Flower Remedies are available in tincture bottles and may be taken orally in drops. Generally, 3 drops of a chosen tincture or tinctures are added to 3 ounces of water, and sipped three times a day. I've found that anywhere from one to seven remedies can be taken at one time. Also, the protocol can be changed as frequently as is deemed necessary. The Bach Flower Remedies can also be EMT tested like any supplement and evaluated for dose, frequency, and duration (see chapter 6).

Essential Oils

Research has shown that human cells begin mutating when electromagnetic frequency drops below 62 MHz. Disease manifests between 38 and 58 MHz, and the electromagnetic vibrational wave frequency at death has been measured at 10–20 MHz. Interestingly, the frequencies produced by the lowest negative mental states are actually lower than those of disease and only slightly higher than the frequencies at death. In the mid-twentieth century, noted researcher Royal Raymond Rife determined that the average electromagnetic frequency of a healthy human body is between 62 and 72 MHz. Therefore, any energetic influences capable of elevating low human frequencies should be considered potentially healing influences.

Aromatherapist Valory Rose describes how the frequencies are measured. "During his work with plants, soil, and water in his agricultural projects, Bruce Tainio of Tainio Technology invented and built a machine called a BT3 Frequency Monitoring System. This device—modified and perfected over years—used a highly sensitive sensor to measure bio-electrical frequencies of plant nutrients and essential oils.

"To summarize how it worked—As a Hertzian wave is generated and travels out from its source, it transfers energy to the objects it passes through. The frequency monitor's sensor measures the nano voltage of that wave, using the predominant frequency in the megahertz range, filtering out the lower and higher ranges. The BT3 measures the composite frequency of the vibratory emissions in electrical voltage—MHz—of the elements and enzymes remaining in the oils."[8]

Rose goes on to list some of the essential oil frequencies discovered by Tainio:

Rose: 320 MHz
Lavender: 118 MHz
Myrrh: 105 MHz
Blue chamomile: 105 MHz
Juniper: 98 MHz

Aloe: 96 MHz
Sandalwood: 96 MHz
Angelica: 85 MHz
Peppermint: 78 MHz
Galbanum: 56 MHz
Basil: 52 MHz

Essential oils are concentrated, plant-based liquids that contain distilled extractions of volatile agents that emit strong fragrances. These aromatic oils have been effectively used to reduce stress, anxiety, mental fatigue, and depression since the late twelfth century. Their dynamic medicinal quality is activated through the sense of smell, or olfaction.

"The sense of smell was one of the earliest, well-developed senses to rise from the evolution of animals," writes aromatherapist Shanti Dechen. "Olfaction is the process of the brain perceiving odor. It is utilized to detect odors of food, enemies, territory, and the opposite sex. In humans and animals, olfaction evokes emotional reactions that result in strong behavior changes. The limbic system is where our memories, instincts, and vital functions are controlled and processed. . . . The sense of smell registers at the subconscious level; it is connected to the limbic system, which regulates the sensory and motor activities. The limbic system contains at least 10,000 times more information than the senses of sight, taste, and touch combined. Stimulation of the limbic system sends signals to the visceral behavioral mechanisms of the autonomic nervous system (ANS), which affects digestion, sexual, and emotional behavior.

"Airborne molecules travel into the nose, passing through the nasal mucosa in the upper regions of the nose. These molecules then travel through minute holes in the cribriform plate of the ethmoid bone in the olfactory bulb of the cranial nerve before entering directly into the limbic system of the brain."[9]

When we inhale these powerful oils, their molecular presence is gathered up by our olfactory receptors, which carry limbic impulses to the autonomic nervous system, which then trigger hormonal secretions and neurotransmissions throughout the entire body.

Once the oil's olfactory influence elicits limbic and hormonal responses, emotions are strongly affected. Some of the emotional responses activated by essential oils have been shown to alter appetite. According to research performed by Dr. Bryan Raudenbush of Wheeling Jesuit University, those subjects who sniffed essence of peppermint oil consumed nearly 300 fewer calories from saturated fat, or 23 percent fewer calories based on 1,800 calories a day, for seven days.[10]

"Smelling your way thin may sound too good to be true," writes Dr. Michelle Schoffro Cook, "but according to exciting research at Niigata University School of Medicine in Japan, certain scents trigger weight loss. According to the study published in *Experimental Biology and Medicine*, the smell of grapefruit and lemon activates the body's ability to burn fat while suppressing further weight gain.

"Other research at the Department of Nursing at the Wonkwang Health Science [University] in Korea found that abdominal massage with specific essential oils reduced belly fat in postmenopausal women."[11]

For our purposes, there are two primary methods for delivering essential oils into the human body:

1. Inhalation—breathed in
2. Topical application—massaged in

For the WHD, I've selected my five favorite aromatherapy essential oil blends to support your total wellness and weight loss plan:

1. Myrtle is often indicated to support hypothyroid and to balance negative emotions.
2. Clove is also commonly used to stimulate underactive thyroid.
3. Nutmeg is especially beneficial for hormonal balancing. This oil provides great support for the adrenal and thyroid glands.
4. Palmarosa is extremely beneficial for stress, acute anxiety, and digestive problems.
5. Lavender is very soothing and relaxing for mind and body. It is also noted for its ability to balance thyroid metabolism, and to help with fluid retention.

Buy these five essential oils in therapeutic grade. Dab one drop of each, in turn, on your finger so that you can apply one oil at a time directly to the base of your throat (thyroid gland). Gently massage the oils together into your tissues at the base of your throat, twice daily, morning and evening.

CHAPTER 8

THE WHD EIGHT-STEP "TRANSFORMACTION" PLAN

I love words, and I really love to formulate new words. I recently fashioned the word "transformaction," and here's a little of what I had in mind. The word "action" refers to energy. Action may be powerful, but it typically comes in short bursts. The word "transformation," on the other hand, indicates a shift that results in a lasting change. One definition of my word "transformaction" then might be: a powerful shift that brings about lasting change.

Every one of us knows what it means to make a resolution, only to hit a wall. We all know well the frustration of wanting and trying to change, only to fail. One of the reasons for this is that the source of our action isn't rooted deeply enough. Instead of planting the seeds of our resolution in our heart, soul, spirit, and quantum mind, we fruitlessly plant them within the will of our ego.

The WHD provides you with the following eight-step transformaction plan to help you flow through a powerful shift that's certain to bring about positive, inexhaustible results. This eight-step action plan is designed to take you deeper, so as to ensure both dramatic changes and lasting effects.

The first and second steps of your eight-step plan are "energy-based" steps. They present you with powerful mind exercises created to help you marshal greater manifest energy—to help transform your material life beyond limitation. The remaining six action steps are "matter-based" steps, intended to help you to better organize and motivate yourself as they empower you to keep your higher intentions engaged for long-term action and attainment.

1. CREATE A SACRED PLACE FROM WHICH TO MANIFEST YOUR MIRACLES

I once visited an aging relative in a nursing home and encountered an experience I've not forgotten since. As I accompanied my loved one into the cafeteria, my attention was immediately drawn to an intriguing man who was sitting directly across from us. The aide who was seated beside us explained that during his younger years, the man had been a master luthier, world renowned for his rare, handcrafted violins. He appeared deeply troubled as he sat there with his head in his hands. I could hear him faintly repeating a haunting phrase over and over: "Oh, the noise of the world." The feelings that prompted his words were unnerving—they struck me deeply.

I could clearly sense his deep frustration as he labored to find some semblance of peace of mind. I watched as the poor man struggled mightily to mute the vapid cacophony of clanging dishes, disjointed conversations, and manic television audio. The noise of the world was frustrating his attempts to create a sacred place of peace.

We all have sacred places of peace and transcendence deep within, which eclipse our mortal minds—domains of consciousness that enable us to create peace and manifest miracles. If not for the distracting noise of the world, we could effortlessly create our sacred places, and miracles would be commonplace.

Your first transformaction step is to create a sacred place from which to manifest your miracles. The following exercise will help you do just that. In order to get started, you'll have to stop! Step out of the "now" moment you're in, and go all the way to the end vision of your desired goal. This sacred journey must begin at the end. By ushering your way to the end of your desired vision you'll gain access to the map of how best to get there. Then, you'll easily be able to get there by simply walking backward in your mind.

Close your eyes and visualize yourself having completed the successful achievement of your desired goal, captured in a single still-life picture within your mind's eye. Include as many sensory details as you possibly can. If, for example, your ultimate desired goal is to lose fifty pounds, then envision yourself in your mind as being fifty pounds lighter. Be sure to accompany your vision with an array of embellishing sights, sounds, smells, and feelings. For example, you might envision yourself healthy and fit, walking a beautiful beach on a radiant, sun-drenched day. Imagine feeling the warm rays blanketing your skin. Imagine hearing the seagulls and pounding surf as you inhale the fragrant salty air. The more vividly you envision the details, the better. These sensory details are referred to as submodalities in the world of neuro-linguistic programming (NLP).

Over the past forty-five years, NLP research has mapped out the human brain and discovered that the greater the sensory richness and diversity of the imagination during any experience, the more likely the mind is to download that experience. Also, the more detailed the submodality development, the deeper the brain will download the memory. The deeper the download, the more empowered the vision is to change your mind's landscape of reality.

Most of us are not aware of it, but the person we are today is mostly the result of submodality downloading. The sum total of all our positive and negative beliefs is directly correlated with the sensory details affixed to our life experiences. Both our functional and dysfunctional realities are largely determined by our unconscious mind. Our conscious mind can process thousands of bits of information per second, but our unconscious mind can process billions of bits of information per second. Unbeknownst to our conscious mind, our unconscious mind takes in and recalls nearly our entire life experience.

NLP research has discovered that much of the unconscious mind's reality-shaping memory is drawn to sensory details. All our devils and our angels are in these details. The important point here is that with the help of submodality visualization, we have the power to eliminate and override any old negative messages that may have repeatedly frustrated our ongoing attempts to reach desired goals. What's more, submodality visualization allows us to embed new positive downloads to replace old negative downloads, so as to enable us to finally reach our desired goals.

So: stop, step out of the "now" moment you're in, and go all the way to the end vision of your desired goal. This visualization exercise needn't take more than a minute or two, but it should be repeated with great frequency. Each time you return to this sacred place of miracles in your mind, you'll add another brick to the foundation of your dreams.

2. GO TO THE END AND WALK BACK TO WHERE YOU ARE

Now it's time for the second transformaction step. With the help of visualization, you've already arrived at your final destination. Now, to take the next step, you'll have to go to the end and walk back to where you are, in your mind. Every journey has a beginning, a middle, and an end. "Go to the end and walk back to where you are" is a visualization exercise that asks you to envision yourself moving in reverse direction—from the end of your miracle journey to the middle, and finally back to the beginning. This is the perfect antidote for being stuck before ever getting out of the starting gate. Far too many fail to attain their desired goals before they even get started, because they just don't know where to begin.

Unlike the first visualization exercise, "Go to the end and walk back" doesn't call for graphic submodalities. Instead, it asks you to generally envision yourself moving in reverse from the successful achievement of your goal, to the middle phase of hard work and process, and finally back to the beginning jump-off point. By repeatedly going to the end of our dreams and reversing direction we clear timeless pathways to our future dreams.

Once again close your eyes and imagine yourself looking down at your feet standing firmly on the square of your miracle achievement. As you're looking down you notice two additional squares. The square closest to you represents the middle of your success journey, and the square just beyond it represents the beginning.

Picture yourself in your mind's eye taking one giant step, landing both feet firmly on the square that represents the middle of your journey. While standing on your middle journey square, focus your attention on embracing the process.

Observe your dedication to the hard work demanded of you—feel your un-yielding will as you envision yourself pushing through and getting traction. In short, imagine yourself feeling a sense of true satisfaction knowing that your efforts are at last paying off. You needn't take more than a minute to focus on this vision.

Moving on, imagine yourself taking one more giant step so that both feet have landed firmly on the third and final space, the beginning journey square. While on the beginning journey square, it's important for you to focus on the enthu-siasm and confidence necessary to begin your miracle journey of attainment. Once again, this step does not require any vivid visualization, or submodality input. It is intended to uproot all the fear, doubt, and lack of confidence that have repeatedly undermined your enthusiasm to achieve. The beginning journey part of this exercise gives you the opportunity to embed a powerful new message in your unconscious mind, enabling you to finally overcome the obstacles that have long sabotaged your desire to attain your prized goals.

3. TAKE THREE GIANT STEPS

Now that you've taken your two "energy-based" transformaction steps toward your desired goals, it's time to take your first tangible, "matter-based" steps. Before you go anywhere, you need to know where you're going. So sit down, collect your thoughts, and think clearly about the task you are about to select as your first real, tangible action step toward your desired goal.

Your first action step should be a baby step. That is to say, it should be doable, but it should also be challenging in a way that gets the attention of your nervous system. If you don't feel at least a little nervous when thinking about this task, then it's the wrong choice. There's got to be some tension in the steps you take toward your desired goal, or there'll be no transformactional growth. There's a great line that comes to mind here, spoken by Luisa Rey, a character in the novel *Cloud Atlas*: "You have to do whatever you can't not do." Every time we impose our will over our fear, we create a new level of personal power.

Next, design a three-part, three-step map. The three parts of your map should include the where, when, and how of your first three tangible steps. So take some time to sit down with paper and pen, or use the notepad on your smartphone. Record the date, and then write down your answers in three separate categories for each of your three steps:

For Step 1, Step 2, and Step 3:

1. What I'm going to do:
2. When I'm going to do it:
3. How I'm going to get it done:

The first part—"what"—asks you to specifically define the task that you've selected to physically initiate your transformaction plan. Your first step should be a baby step, like waking up early tomorrow morning and taking a brisk three-mile walk. Remember, these tasks should start off relatively undemanding and gradually build in their degree of challenge in accordance with your achievement growth. The key is to take one step toward your highest goal every day! Numbers two and three on your map are equally self-explanatory. They are merely designed to make your self-empowerment journey more conceptual.

Your three-part, three-step map should be continually updated as you evolve through your goal achievement process. Choose your challenges wisely and take your steps fearlessly. To quote author George Addair: "Everything you've ever wanted is on the other side of fear!"

4. FAIL TO SUCCEED

Words have power. Words like "love," "death," "ecstasy," and "cancer" all have the power to evoke strong emotions that have powerful effects on our entire being via our nervous system. Words derive their meaning and power from belief. This step of our action plan is about changing our belief about word meaning and power. After all, whether we choose to accept or to alter the meaning and power of words is a matter of choice. For example, after centuries of having a negative connotation, the words "wicked" and "bad" have suddenly been assigned a totally opposite, positive meaning by pop culture. Perhaps no word in the English dictionary has greater meaning and power than the word "failure." It's a damning and often disabling power that's laid many a goal to waste. So what's the story, I'm sure you're asking yourself, with the header of this action step?

"Fail to succeed" looks crazy, but you must admit, it did get your nervous system's attention. This header is intended to teach us that if we are to succeed, we must learn to do so through failure. We must come to understand failure as an agent of success. We've been taught to fear and loathe failure, and to celebrate success, as if they were two diametric opposites. In truth, the greatest secret to high achievement comes with the understanding that success and failure are opposite parts of one whole.

Ancient Chinese sages often spoke of the importance of understanding what they called the mutual compatibility of opposition. The tai chi circle, or yin/yang symbol, serves as a visual metaphor for this philosophy, as it depicts two polar opposites appearing side by side, each dependent upon the other to create wholeness. This philosophy represents an extreme departure from contemporary Western culture. In the West, we've been taught to think of opposition as adversarial. In the East, it's believed that even the tension that emerges from the forces of opposition is sacred. In accordance with this philosophy, it is understood that there are only blessings or lessons, and if properly understood, the lessons learned can be turned into blessings. And so it is with success and failure. Only our failures can teach us the lessons that only we can turn into our blessings.

In this transformaction step you artistically fashion an image of the tai chi circle. In the predominantly black side of the circle write the word "SUCCESS" in bold white lettering. In the predominantly white side of the circle write the word "FAILURE" in bold black lettering. Next, print at least six copies of your mandala. Place these images in strategic spots where you're bound to see one at all times throughout your day. Tape one to your bedroom mirror, and another to your refrigerator door. Put one in your car. Keep one at work. Don't let them out of your sight until you know that you've truly gotten the message. You will know when you have.

Note: The word *mandala* is a five-thousand-year-old Sanskrit word meaning "circle." Mandalas have long been considered spiritual symbols of power that can assist in bringing forth transformation, wisdom, and unity.

5. UNCONDITIONALIZE YOUR MIND

The truth is, it's never really been about being too tired, too busy, too early, too late, too dark, too bright, too fast, too slow, too hot, too cold, too wet, too windy, too sunny, too cloudy, too icy, or anything else. It's always been about fear. In fact, it's about being so fearful of "the great unknown" associated with failure and success that you've developed a self-protective defense tactic that keeps you safe from the risk of participation. If your road to success is blocked by an unending list of conditions, it means you're working overtime in the control room.

This transformaction step on your path to goal attainment is actually more of a quantum leap. It demands that you make the decision to leap over the internment walls of your self-limiting fears. I've always embraced the belief that "it's not about conditions, it's about decisions."

Change is very difficult for us. Making the decision to meet change head-on can be paralyzing. We all have a tendency to settle into our comfort zones, because they represent a known history of safety and predictability. Whenever our safety and predictability are in question, alarms are triggered in our brain that put our entire body into a state of "fight or flight." Our brain is naturally wired for primal fear, in the region between the amygdala and the right prefrontal cortex. Our primal fear wiring represents an important part of our natural defense system, designed for the protection and survival of our species. All this powerful brain machinery networks its way to the far reaches of our unconscious mind. The first time our primitive ancestors touched fire, their primal fear mechanism instantly associated that pain in the brain's amygdala and right prefrontal cortex, where it was then recorded in their unconscious mind. Once the pain experience makes its way into the unconscious mind, it can never be forgotten. From that time on, the mere mention of fire would elicit the same stress response. And so it is with us whenever we contemplate the unknown possibilities of the next potential failure.

The good news here is that all that primal wiring between our brain and our unconscious mind is not hardwired. It's neuroplastic, meaning that it can be rewired. Neuroscience has discovered that the human brain was naturally designed to be neurologically rewired and reformatted. Perhaps the best news is that all this rewiring and reformatting can be accomplished by simply changing our inner dialogue.

To engage the process of unconditionalizing your mind and overcoming your fear of the unpredictability of change, you'll have to start listening to your dialogue. Devote one whole day of your life to tuning in to your inner and outer dialogue. Listen to the words and phrases that you most commonly tend to speak, both internally and externally, and listen especially intently to the energy and emotion behind your words. Does the energy of your spoken words reveal a positive or negative spirit? Also, listen closely to the words spoken by those with whom you spend most of your time. Listen to the energy behind the words most frequently spoken by your significant other, your family, your closest friends, and your work associates. It won't be long before you start to get a clear picture of why you've become so fearfully conditionalized. Whether we achieve or we fail to succeed, it all begins with our words.

We are all either right-brain or left-brain prefrontal dominant. Right prefrontal types tend to be more emotionally fear based, and therefore more inclined to self-limiting conditionalization. Upon contemplation of taking on any great challenge, the inner dialogue of the right-prefrontal-dominant type is likely "I can't because I'm too tired/too busy; it's too early/too late." On the other hand, left-prefrontal-dominant types are more likely to hear the inner voice of their inspired self, encouraging them with confidence-building words and phrases.

Our words represent cause and effect. They both reflect and create our mental states. Research has proven beyond a shadow of a doubt that by merely changing our dialogue, we can change our neural pathways. Research continues to show that words alone alter brain chemistry. Positive words elicit a positive neurological effect and negative words have a negative effect. Words are associated with meaning. Meaning generates strong emotional energy, which has a profound effect on our entire nervous system.

The salient message of this transformaction step is this: if you truly wish to succeed, you'll first have to change your nervous system by replacing all your fear-based words with words of love and happiness. Instead of "I can't achieve my desired goal because I'm too tired, busy, early, late, etc.," you'll have to tell yourself, "I will achieve my desired goal irrespective of any and all conditions, because I'm empowered by all the love and happiness that I continually create."

The best brain-reformatting results can be attained simply by devoting four minutes every morning and afternoon to the repetition of a sensationalized, positive incantation. I say "sensationalized" because your nervous system will only be drawn into the process if it hears words not commonly spoken. Exaggerated mantras like "I am a genius" or "I am the master of the universe" will more than suffice. Remember, your brain's neurology doesn't know or care about accuracy or truth. Your words don't have to be honest or accurate. They simply have to be positive. Don't forget to rehearse your positive mantras for four minutes, twice a day. Feel free to change them up from time to time, and remember to keep up a steady flow of positive self-talk throughout your day. Take charge, and unconditionalize your mind with the reformatting power of your words!

6. PLACE FREQUENT CALLS TO YOUR "SOURCE" HOTLINE

We're always talking to ourselves. As the days of our lives go on, we ponder, we problem solve, and we reminisce within the inner recesses of our minds. Our incessant dialogue with ourselves goes on and on ad infinitum. In fact, the thoughts we think—one thousand to three thousand thoughts per minute—contribute mightily to our busy internal dialogue. So there's a whole lot of chatter going on deep within us. But the all-important question is—exactly who's talking to whom?

In the earlier chapters of this book, a significant assertion was put forth regarding our having two selves. With that in mind, let's assume we're all composed of a higher and a lower self. Let's further imagine our higher self as being imbued with innate wisdom, while our lower self is in need of whatever wisdom it can get. So, when you're listening to your inner voices throughout the day, do you know which self you're taking direction from? Is your lower self doing most of the talking? Are you even aware of the fact that you have access to innate sage advice from your higher self anytime you want it? It's all a matter of how conscious you are. Just think—by merely being aware, you can gain access to an innate stream of consciousness within your mind. To my way of thinking, there's no better place for you to obtain good, sound advice. That's precisely what this action step involves.

In this action step you create a direct hotline to your higher self. It is really quite simple—all that's required is your commitment to ongoing mindfulness. You already talk to yourself all day, every day. This action step suggests that you do it more consciously, so that you're able to clearly determine the source of the information. In time, after you've mastered the discernment, you'll be able to tap into your higher self with consistency and reliability. We all need guidance as we progress through our transformactional evolution. There's nothing quite like having direct access to a divine hotline.

7. BE LEAVING YOUR MIRACLES

It's one thing to believe in miracles; it's another thing altogether to be leaving miracles in your wake. During this time of shifting consciousness, increasing numbers among us are routinely performing miracles. This transformaction step is about turning on our miracle-making machinery. In order for us to tap into our miracle-manifesting potential we must first come to fully understand the vivifying power of belief.

Belief activates both passive and active aspects of our nature. Most of us remain stuck in old passive-belief programming, daring not to believe because of disappointment or skepticism. Passive believers do believe but only sometimes. They are generally willing to believe, but only when their material senses and their logical conscience permit them. Passive believers need lots of reassurance before they invest. Their apprehension casts a wet blanket on their magical fire. Active believers are more willing to push through skepticism and cultural pressure. By letting go of these diminishing forces, we activate a level of faith that unleashes the supernatural energy that engages our manifest power. Belief in the face of uncertainty is exactly what it takes to power up our miracle machinery.

Something otherworldly happens to us when we believe. By projecting skepticism, we may be operating from a place of self-protection and good discernment, but we also lose access to our miracle-making power. When we believe, we flip the "miracle-making" switch.

The best way to strengthen our belief in miracles is to learn to believe in ourselves. The best way to believe in ourselves is to engage in action. I'm sure that somewhere near where you live there's a children's hospital, a soup kitchen, an orphanage, or some such place that's waiting for you to take part in a miracle. It's time for you to transcend limitation with action. Give of yourself where it is most needed and watch miracles unfold right before your eyes.

8. AFFIRM THAT YOU ARE A MAKER OF MIRACLES

We are the thoughts that emerge from our minds. Our state of mind manifests our relative reality. Our one thousand to three thousand thoughts per minute flow forth from five different reservoirs within our mind:

1. Negative unconscious—negative and unaware of it
2. Positive unconscious—positive and unaware of it
3. Negative conscious—negative and aware of it
4. Positive conscious—positive and aware of it
5. Superconscious—positive, aware, and fully in control of it

Each of our reservoirs produces a different state of mind. Unfortunately, according to neuroscience, our minds spend most of their time in the negative unconscious state. In fact, research tells us that we are spending approximately 96 percent of our time unconsciously in the negative thought state. Therefore, we're walking around ruminating about the worst possible outcomes all day without being conscious of it. What's worse, brain science also now tells us that, unbeknownst to us, we inadvertently slip in and out of trance states hundreds of times per day.

Trance states are altered brain-wave states that produce a "spaced out" effect, much like when we gaze out a window into the distance with some degree of disconnect. Trance states are extremely fertile mind states, conducive to the planting of transformational thoughts that can radically alter behavior. Behavioral change through hypnosis is an example of how trance can access our deepest unconscious mind. So you might say that by unconsciously hypnotizing ourselves hundreds of times a day, we're reinforcing thoughts, beliefs, and behaviors that exert a powerful influence on our perception of reality.

When you then consider the fact that 96 percent of our existing thought patterns are unconsciously negative, the picture starts to look very troubling. In fact, many of us are unwittingly embedding negative thoughts deep into the innermost recesses of our unconscious mind all day, every day. Imagine how many millions of us are lying in bed falling asleep to the news every night. As we're lying there half-asleep, in trance, we're reinforcing all of our most negative and fearful forebodings. All this doesn't leave us much room for positive conscious and superconscious thinking.

Positive conscious thinking represents our good intentions—like wanting to lose weight, to be fit, and to be healthy. The only thing here is, no matter how consciously positive or determined our intentions are to lose weight, to be fit, and to be healthy, they're heavily outgunned by the neurology of our negative unconscious mind. Thus, it's easy to see why there aren't as many miracles being manifested as there could be.

The superconscious mind is the miracle-making domain of the mind. The concept of superconsciousness relates back to the idea of paying attention to what we're paying attention to. Awareness of our awareness affords us the power to change our perception. It's like being both the lead actor and the director of your life movie. So consider the possibilities here. Most of us are chronically negative and unaware of it; some of us are consciously positive—but only until the chronic negativity returns; and few if any of us are locked into a superconscious flow. One more important point here: each of these states of mind represents a choice. Choosing to take superconscious control of our mind can be transformational. It's where miracles are born.

There is a simple but powerful affirmation exercise in the Whole Health Diet that I would like to share with you now as you take your final action step. This step is designed to switch you over to superconscious dominance.

This affirmation exercise is all about you speaking directly to yourself. More to the point, it's about your superconscious soul self speaking directly to your unconscious mortal self. This should be done standing completely nude in front of a mirror. It is recommended that you stare deeply into the pupils of your own eyes in order to align directly with your soul self. You'll be reading from a scripted monologue while still maintaining intermittent eye contact in the mirror.

Imagine that as you read the words of the scripted monologue, your mortal voice has been given over to your soul and that your mortal ears are listening to your soul's immortal voice. So now, as you prepare to connect with your soul, take three slow and deep breaths. Then position yourself in front of the mirror and begin reading the following:

"I am who you are. Throughout your eternity of lessons and blessings, I have always been within you and I forever shall so remain. I am forever silently observing and assisting you. I remain within you even when you think you're alone. My love for you is unconditional, and I will remain here for you anytime you need me. I am your source of infinite light, divine inspiration, and universal transcendence. It is I who makes you the miracle maker that you are. Anytime you desire to reach beyond your mortal grasp, I will be here to empower you. I'd like to remind you that you are always far greater and far more powerful than any of your mortal challenges. There is nothing in this world that you cannot overcome. You are immortal. I am the eyes and voice of your soul. We are as one, for I am in you as you are in me. Go now and know that you have been blessed to perform miracles. Remember, you need only believe in your own soul."

ACKNOWLEDGMENTS

Monique Miller-McCarthy—Illustrations

Bill Wenzel—Graphics

Joel Price, PhD—Technical Support

Andrew Yackira—Guidance and Production

NOTES

Chapter 1: Overweight, Obese, and Dying to Be Transformed

1. www.who.int/mediacentre/fctsheetn311/updated aug 2014./fctsheet311.www .who.int/updatedaug2014.

2. F. B. Hu, W. C. Willet, T. Li et al., "Adiposity as Compared with Physical Activity in Predicting Mortality Among Women," *New England Journal of Medicine* 351, no 26 (2004): 2694–703.

3. Centers for Disease Control and Prevention, "Obesity and Overweight," June 2, 2015, www.cdc.gov/nchs/fastats/obesity-overweight.htm.

4. Sarah C. Walpole, David Prieto-Merino, Phil Edwards et al., "The Weight of Nations: An Estimation of Adult Human Biomass," BMC Public Health 12 (2012), p. 439; http:www.biomedcentral.com/1471-2458/12/439.

5. Sherry Rau, "Is Fat the New Normal?" WebMD, January 26, 2010, www.webmd .com/diet/obesity/is-fat-the-new-normal.

6. "Overweight in Children," American Heart Association, August 17, 2015, http:// www.heart.org/HEARTORG/GettingHealthy/Overweight-in-Children_ UCM_304054_Article.jsp

7. M. R. Lowe, T. V. Kral, and K. Miller-Kovach, "Weight-Loss Maintenance 1, 2 and

5 Years After Successful Completion of a Weight-Loss Programme," *British Journal of Nutrition* 99, no. 4 (2008): 925–30.

8. Das Wesen der Materie [The Nature of Matter], speech at Florence, Italy (1944) (from Archiv zur Geschichte der Max-Planck-Gesellschaft, Abt. Va, Rep. 11 Planck, Nr. 1797.

Chapter 2: The Heart of the Matter

1. David Hawkins, *Power vs. Force: The Hidden Determinants of Human Behavior* (Carlsbad, CA: Hay House, 2002).
2. Lisa Firestone, "What's Behind Emotional Overeating?" *Psychology Today* (blog), May 8, 2012. https://www.psychologytoday.com/blog/compassion-matters/201205/whats-behind-emotional-overeating.
3. David Vanata, American Dietetic Nutrition Conference and Expo, October 2008.
4. John Bradshaw, *Healing the Shame That Binds You* (Houston: Health Communications, 1988).
5. Mara Tyler, "Food Addiction," Healthline, July 7, 2014, http://www.healthline.com/health/addiction/food#Overview1.
6. Emmett Fox, *Find and Use Your Inner Power* (New York: HarperCollins, 1937).
7. Kahlil Gibran, *The Prophet* (New York: Knopf, 1923).

Chapter 3: The Chemistry That Governs Calorie-Burning Energy

1. Byron J. Richards and Mary Guignon Richards, *Mastering Leptin* (Minneapolis: Wellness Resources, 2005).
2. Ibid.
3. Ibid.
4. Ibid.
5. N. Boqué, R. de la Iglesia, A. L. de la Garza et al., "Prevention of Diet-Induced Obesity by Apple Polyphenols in Wistar Rats Through Regulation of Adipocyte Gene Expression and DNA Methylation Patterns," *Molecular Nutrition and Food Research* 57, no. 8 (2013): 1473–78.
6. K. W. Williams, T. Liu, X. Kong et al., "Xbp1s in Pomc Neurons Connects ER Stress

with Energy Balance and Glucose Homeostasis," *Cell Metabolism* 20, no. 3 (2014): 471–82.

7. David L. Watts, *Trace Elements and Other Essential Nutrients* (Dallas: Trace Elements Inc., 1995), p. 1.

8. National Institutes of Health, "Vitamin D Fact Sheet for Health Professionals," November 10, 2014, https://ods.od.nih.gov/factsheets/VitaminD-HealthProfessional.

9. Nathan Seppa, "Link Between Obesity and Vitamin D Clarified," *ScienceNews*, February 5, 2013, https://www.sciencenews.org/article/link-between-obesity-and-vitamin-d-clarified.

10. C. Mason, L. Xiao, I. Imayama et. al., "Effects of Weight Loss on Serum Vitamin D in Postmenopausal Women," *American Journal of Clinical Nutrition* 94, no. 1 (2014): 95–103.

11. M. Chondronikola, E. Volpi, C. Porter et al., "Brown Adipose Tissue Improves Whole-Body Glucose Homeostasis and Insulin Sensitivity in Humans," *Diabetes* 63, no. 12 (2014): 4089–99.

12. J. C. Ratliff, J. Barber, L. Palmese et al., "Association of Prescription H1 Antihistamine Use with Obesity: Results from the National Health and Nutrition Examination Survey," *Obesity* 18, no. 12 (2010): 2398–2400.

13. C. K. Martin, H. Han, S. D. Anton et al., "Effect of Valproic Acid on Body Weight, Food Intake, Physical Activity and Hormones: Results of a Randomized Controlled Trial," *Journal of Psychopharmacology* 23, no. 7 (2009): 814–25.

14. "Vintage Ad #2,270: Without Chemicals, Life Itself Would Be Impossible," Flickr photo, posted by "Jamie," May 15, 2013, https://www.flickr.com/photos/jbcurio/8740859605.

15. D. Melzer, N. Rice, M. H. Depledge et al., "Association Between Serum Perfluorooctanoic Acid (PFOA) and Thyroid Disease in the U.S. National Health and Nutrition Examination Survey," *Environmental Health Perspectives* 118, no. 5 (2010): 686–92.

16. J. D. Meeker and K. K. Ferguson, "Relationship Between Urinary Phthalate and Bisphenol A Concentrations and Serum Thyroid Measures in U.S. Adults and Adolescents from the National Health and Nutrition Examination Survey (NHANES) 2007–2008," *Environmental Health Perspectives* 119 (2011): 1396–1402.

Chapter 4: The Whole Health Diet Primer

1. National Prevention, Health Promotion, and Public Health Council, 2014 *Annual Status Report* (Washington, DC: U.S. Department of Health and Human Services, Office of the Surgeon General, 2014), http://www.surgeongeneral.gov/priorities/prevention/2014-npc-status-report.pdf.

2. Julie Miller Jones, "Food Additives," Food and Drug Administration, 1990.

3. "Farm to Fork: Our Toxic Food System," Healthy Child Healthy World, http://www.healthychild.org/farm-to-fork-our-toxic-food-system/.

4. Christina Sarich, "Europe Bans American Apples—Too Toxic to Eat," Global-Research, June 17, 2014, http://www.globalresearch.ca/europe-bans-american-apples-too-toxic-to-eat/5387379.

5. W. Holtcamp, "Obesogens: An Environmental Link to Obesity," *Environmental Health Perspectives* 120, no. 2 (2012): a62–a68.

6. Jason Cody and Janet Osuch, "Exposure to Insecticide May Play Role in Obesity Epidemic Among Some Women," Michigan State University, March 19, 2009, http://msutoday.msu.edu/news/2009/exposure-to-insecticide-may-play-role-in-obesity-epidemic-among-some-women/.

7. Stephen Perrine and Heather Hurlock, "Fat Epidemic Linked to Chemicals Run Amok," *NBCNews.com*, March 8, 2010, http://www.nbcnews.com/id/35315651/ns/health-diet_and_nutrition/#.Vf3_K5fPw_w.

8. W. S. Goldner, D. P. Sandler, F. Yu et al., "Pesticide Use and Thyroid Disease Among Women in the Agricultural Health Study," *American Journal of Epidemiology* 171, no. 4 (2010): 455–64.

9. Ibid.

10. "Dirty Dozen: EWG's 2015 Shopper's Guide to Pesticides in Produce," Environmental Working Group, http://www.ewg.org/foodnews/dirty_dozen_list.php; "Clean Fifteen: EWG's 2015 Shopper's Guide to Pesticides in Produce," Environmental Working Group, http://www.ewg.org/foodnews/clean_fifteen_list.php.

11. J. Kling, "*JAMA* Study Casts Cloud over Biologic Safety," *Nature Biotechnology* 27, no. 1 (2009): 11–12.

1 2. E. Giovannucci, "Insulin-Like Growth Factor-1 and Binding Protein-3 and Risk of Cancer," *Hormone Research* 51, Suppl. 3 (1999): 34–41.

13. J. S. de Vendômois, F. Roullier, D. Cellier et al., "A Comparison of the Effects of Three GM Corn Varieties on Mammalian Health," *International Journal of Biological Sciences* 5, no. 7 (2009): 706–26.

14. Irina V. Ermakova, "Influence of Genetically Modified Soya on the Birth-Weight and Survival of Rat Pups: Preliminary Study," Institute of Higher Nervous Activity and Neurophysiology, Russian Academy of Sciences, October 10, 2005.

15. Arild S. Foss, "Growing Fatter on a GM Diet," *ScienceNordic*, July 17, 2012, http://sciencenordic.com/growing-fatter-gm-diet.

16. Emily Main, "Are GMOs Making You Fat?" *Prevention*, August 20, 2012, http://www.prevention.com/food/healthy-eating-tips/gmo-foods-linked-weight-gain.

17. Roddy Scheer and Doug Moss, "Dirt Poor: Have Fruits and Vegetables Become Less Nutritious?" *Scientific American*, April 27, 2011, http://www.scientificamerican.com/article/soil-depletion-and-nutrition-loss/.

18. Hilary Parker, "A Sweet Problem: Princeton Researchers Find That High-Fructose Corn Syrup Prompts Considerably More Weight Gain," Princeton University, March 22, 2010, http://www.princeton.edu/main/news/archive/S26/91/22K07/.

19. Nicholas Perricone, *The Perricone Prescription* (New York: HarperCollins, 2002), 40.

20. Bryan Walsh, "Eat Butter," *Time*, June 23, 2014.

21. S. E. Steck, A. M. Chalecki, P. Miller et al., "Conjugated Linoleic Acid Supplementation for Twelve Weeks Increases Lean Body Mass in Obese Humans," *Journal of Nutrition* 137, no. 5 (2007): 1188–93.

22. J. M. Gaullier, J. Halse, K. Høye et al., "Conjugated Linoleic Acid Supplementation for 1 y Reduces Body Fat Mass in Healthy Overweight Humans," *American Journal of Clinical Nutrition* 79, no. 6 (2004): 1118–25.

Chapter 5: A Matter of Energy

1. Pam Grout, *E-Squared* (New York: Hay House, 2013), 1–2.

2. Stuart Hameroff and Roger Penrose, "Orchestrated Reduction of Quantum Coherence

in Brain Microtubules: A Model for Consciousness," *Mathematics and Computers in Simulation* 40 (1996): 453–80.

3. Peter Baksa, "Can Thoughts Make Things Happen?" *The Way the Universe Works* (blog), October 18, 2011, http://blog.peterbaksa.com/post/11632947492/can-thoughts -makethings-happen. Oct. 2011.

4. "Imagination More Important Than Knowledge?" *I Give You Papyrus* (blog), March 2015, http://prashjay.tumblr.com/post/116720379110/imagination-more-import ant-than-knowledge.

5. V. K. Ranganathan, V. Siemionow, J. Z. Liu et al., "From Mental Power to Muscle Power—Gaining Strength by Using the Mind," *Neuropsychologia* 42, no. 7 (2004): 944–56.

6. E. M. Shackell and L. G. Standing, "Mind over Matter: Mental Training Increases Physical Strength," North *American Journal of Psychology* 9, no. 1 (2007): 189–200.

7. Sharon Begley, "The Brain: How the Brain Rewires Itself," *Time*, January 19, 2007.

8. C. K. Morewedge, Y. E. Huh, and J. Vosgerau, "Thought for Food: Imagined Consumption Reduces Actual Consumption," *Science* 330, no. 6010 (2010): 1530–33.

Chapter 6: Our Energy Guidance System (EGS)

1. Kelly Turner, "The Science Behind Intuition," *Psychology Today* (blog), May 20, 2014, https://www.psychologytoday.com/blog/radical-remission/201405/the-science -behind-intuition.

2. Anne T. Denogean, "Mother Knows Best When Guessing Her Baby's Sex," *Tucson Citizen*, September 26, 1998, http://tucsoncitizen.com/morgue2/1998/09/26/ 90790-mother-knows-best-when-guessing-her-baby-s-sex/; Victor Shamas, Amanda Dawson, The Intuition in Pregnancy Study, University of Arizona, 1998.

3. "New Study Further Supports Intuition," HeartMath Institute, October 2, 2010, https://www.heartmath.org/articles-of-the-heart/science-of-the-heart/ new-study-further-supports-intuition/.

4. Mayo Clinic Staff, "Biofeedback: Using Your Mind to Improve Your Health," Mayo Clinic, January 26, 2013, http://www.mayoclinic.org/tests-procedures/biofeedback/ basics/definition/prc-20020004.

Chapter 7: Balancing Metabolism with Energy Medicine

1. Paul F. M. Nogier, *Treatise of Auriculotherapy* (Moulins-les-metz, France: Maison-neuve, 1972).

2. Belinda Weber, "Ear Acupuncture Boosts Weight Loss," *Medical News Today*, December 17, 2013, http://www.medicalnewstoday.com/articles/270158.php; S. Yeo, K. S. Kim, and S. Lim, "Randomised Clinical Trial of Five Ear Acupuncture Points for the Treatment of Overweight People," *Acupuncture in Medicine* 32, no. 2 (2014): 132–38.

3. Richard Gerber, *Vibrational Medicine* (Santa Fe, NM: Bear and Co., 1988), 86.

4. Dana Ullman, "Homeopathic Medicine: Europe's #1 Alternative for Doctors," *HuffPost Healthy Living* (blog), May 3, 2010, http://www.huffingtonpost.com/dana-ullman/homeopathic- medicineeuro_b_402490.html.

5. Ibid.; Dana Ullman, "The Case FOR Homeopathic Medicine: The Historical and Scientific Evidence," *HuffPost Healthy Living* (blog), April 12, 2010, http://www.huffingtonpost.com/dana-ullman/the-case-for-homeopathic_b_451187.html.

6. Colin F. Watson and Jayne L. Watson, *HCG Body for Life: How to Feel Good Naked in 26 Days* (Create Space Independent Publishing Platform, 2010). hcgbodyforlife.com.

7. Edward Bach, *The Essential Writings of Dr Edward Bach* (London: Vermilion, 2005).

8. Valory Rose, "Vibrational Frequency and the Subtle Energy Nature of Essential Oils," BioSpiritual Energy Healing, http://www.biospiritual-energy-healing.com/vibrational-frequency.html.

9. Shanti Dechen, *Clinical Aromatherapy Level I* (Crestone, CO: Aroma Apothecary Healing Arts Academy, 2011).

10. "Peppermint Vapor Studies: NASA and Others," Essential Potions, http://www.femlogic.com/peppermint_study.html.

11. Michelle Schoffro Cook, "Certain Scents Trigger Weight Loss," Care 2, January 16, 2014, http://www.care2.com/greenliving/proven-aromatherapy-for-weight-loss.html.

INDEX